VIRAL REPLICATION

Edited by **German Rosas-Acosta**

Viral Replication
http://dx.doi.org/10.5772/3017
Edited by German Rosas-Acosta

Contributors

Andrés Santos, Jason Chacón, Germán Rosas-Acosta, George Valiakos, Labrini V. Athanasiou, Antonia Touloudi, Vassilis Papatsiros, Vassiliki Spyrou, Liljana Petrovska, Charalambos Billinis, MariaKuttikan Jayalakshmi, Narayanan Kalyanaraman, Ramasamy Pitchappan, S. Chakraborty, B.M. Veeregowda, R. Deb,, B.M. Chandra Naik, Paul J. Hanson, Huifang M. Zhang, Maged Gomaa Hemida, Xin Ye, Ye Qiu, Decheng Yang, Zeinab N. Said, Kouka S. Abdelwahab

Published by InTech

Janeza Trdine 9, 51000 Rijeka, Croatia

Publishing Process Manager Marina Jozipovic
Technical Editor InTech DTP team
Cover InTech Design team

Additional hard copies can be obtained from orders@intechopen.com

Viral Replication, Edited by German Rosas-Acosta
p. cm.
ISBN 978-953-51-1055-2

For EU product safety concerns:
IN TECH d.o.o., Prolaz Marije Krucifikse Kozulić 3, 51000 Rijeka, Croatia,
info@intechopen.com or visit our website at intechopen.com.

Meet the editor

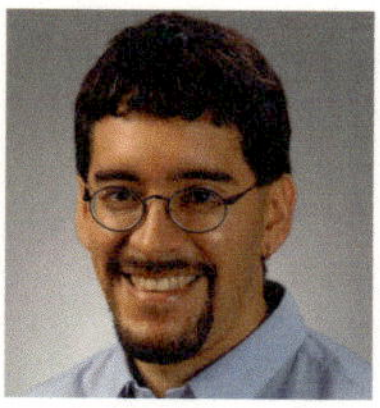

Dr. Germán Rosas-Acosta was born and raised in Colombia, where he graduated from the Universidad de Los Andes with a BS degree in Microbiology. After working for 3 years as research associate at the Instituto de Inmunologia, Hospital San Juan de Dios, he moved to New York City, where he completed his MS and PhD degrees in Biomedical Sciences at the Sackler Institute of Graduate Biomedical Sciences, New York University Medical Center. Dr. Rosas-Acosta went on to perform post-doctoral studies, first at Texas A&M University, and later at the College of Medicine, Texas A&M Health Science Center, where he performed research on the role of SUMO on Papillomavirus infections, under the direction of Dr. Van G. Wilson. Dr. Rosas-Acosta joined The University of Texas at El Paso (UTEP) as an assistant professor in 2007, and his laboratory has played a key role in studying the interactions established between the cellular SUMOylation system and influenza A virus during infection. Dr. Rosas-Acosta's research has been supported by the American Heart Association, the National Institute of General Medical Sciences (NIGMS) and the National Institute of Allergy and Infectious Disease (NIAID), National Institutes of Health, USA.

Contents

Preface

This book is the result of the combined effort of an international panel of experts on different areas of virological research. Therefore, rather than presenting an exhaustive review of a very focused virological area, it provides a collection of in-depth reviews broadly related to the mechanisms of viral replication as applied to various viruses of critical relevance for human or animal disease.

Specifically, this book contains six different chapters.

Chapter one, "Influenza A Virus Multiplication and the Cellular SUMOylation System," summarizes our current knowledge of the mechanisms governing Influenza A transcription and replication, and provides an in depth review of our current knowledge of the interactions established between the cellular SUMOylation system and influenza virus during infection, indicating how knowledge related to this topic may lead to innovative new therapeutic approaches against influenza.

Chapter two, "West Nile Virus: Basic Principles, Replication Mechanism, Immune Response and Important Genetic Determinants of Virulence," provides a thorough review of our current knowledge of the molecular biology of West Nile Virus, with emphasis on its structure, genome, replication cycle, epidemiology, pathogenesis, and the genetic determinants of viral virulence.

Chapter three, "Hepatitis B Virus Genetic Diversity: Disease Pathogenesis," gives a general overview of the molecular biology of Hepatitis B virus, with particular emphasis on its mechanisms of replication, the role played by the different proteins encoded by the virus during its life cycle, viral genotypes and sub-genotypes, and their link with pathogenesis in the outcome of viral infection.

Chapter four, "An Overview of the Immune Evasion Strategies Adopted by Different Viruses With Special Reference to Classical Swine Fever Virus," presents a brief review of the general mechanisms used by viruses to evade the immune responses of their host, with special emphasis on the mechanisms used by Classical Swine Fever Virus.

Chapter five, "Viral Replication Strategies: Manipulation of ER Stress Response Pathways and Promotion of IRES-Dependent Translation," presents an in-depth review of our current knowledge of ER Stress Response Pathway and how viral infection utilizes this pathway to stimulate cap-independent (IRES-dependent) translation. Furthermore, it provides an overview of the different Internal Ribosomal Entry Sites encoded by viruses, their classification, mechanism of action, and how viruses manipulate the cellular environment to enhance their activity.

And chapter six, "Antiviral Replication Agents," gives a general overview of antiviral chemotherapeutic agents currently licensed for clinical used and their mechanisms of action, with emphasis on the viral processes and components targeted by them.

This book is aimed at students, scholars, professors, and investigators who are peripherally related to, or somehow intrigued by, the different areas of virology covered in this book, as well as at those individuals with greater expertise and knowledge in the topics herein presented who may want up-to-date in depth reviews related to such topics.

We expect that, in addition to providing excellent reviews in various exciting areas of virological research, this book will also stimulate the type of scientific discussions and ideas that will result in sustained research efforts not only in the specific areas of research covered in this book, but also in other related areas of biomedical research.

German Rosas-Acosta, PhD.
Border Biomedical Research Center (BBRC), The University of Texas at El Paso (UTEP),
Department of Biological Sciences, The University of Texas at El Paso (UTEP),
USA

Chapter 1

Influenza A Virus Multiplication and the Cellular SUMOylation System

Andrés Santos, Jason Chacón and Germán Rosas-Acosta

Additional information is available at the end of the chapter

http://dx.doi.org/10.5772/54351

> "Medical care was making little difference anyway. Mary Tullidge daughter of Dr. George Tullidge, died twenty-four hours after her first symptoms. Alice Wolowitz, a student nurse at Mount Sinai Hospital, began her shift in the morning, felt sick, and was dead twelve hours later."
>
> "In ten days - *ten days!* - the epidemic had exploded from a few hundred civilian cases and one or two deaths a day to hundreds of thousands ill and hundreds of deaths each day."
>
> Excerpts from Chapter Nineteen, "The Great Influenza" by John. M. Barry.
>
> It is impossible to predict with absolute certainty whether we will ever face another pandemic like that of the 1918 Spanish flu. But nevertheless, we must be prepared to fight it in the event that it might happen. Increasing our knowledge of the molecular biology of the virus is by far the best way to get ready for it. In fact, it might be the only way.
>
> GRA.

1. Introduction

1.1. A coated agent with a fragmented genome: The infectious viral particle of Influenza A Virus

Influenza A virus (IAV), a member of the Orthomyxoviridae [1], is an enveloped, negative-sense, RNA virus that contains a segmented genome composed of eight different viral RNA strands (vRNAs), each coding for one or two different viral proteins [2]. The viral particle is composed of a phospholipid bilayer membrane derived from the plasma membrane of the host, decorated by two single transmembrane domain viral proteins, the hemagglutinin

(HA) and neuraminidase (NA) proteins, and one pore-forming protein, the matrix 2 (M2) ion channel protein [3]. The viral envelope surrounds a relatively irregular viral nucleocapsid formed by the viral matrix (M1) protein, which in turn surrounds eight viral ribonucleoproteins (vRNPs) that appear to be placed in a well organized cylindrical arrangement [4]. Each vRNP is made of a single stranded viral genomic RNA segment covered by numerous copies of the viral nucleoprotein (NP), and a single copy of the viral RNA-dependent RNA-polymerase (RdRp), which is associated to a double stranded RNA structure formed by 12 and 13 complementary nucleotides at the 5' and 3' end regions in each gene segment, respectively. The viral RdRp is a trimeric complex made of single copies of the basic one, basic two, and acid RNA polymerase proteins (referred to as PB1, PB2, and PA, respectively). Also associated to the infectious viral particle is the nuclear export protein (NEP), formerly known as non-structural protein 2 (NS2), a protein involved in the export of vRNPs from the nucleus of infected cells (Reviewed by Nayak et al [5], and Rossman and Lamb [3]) (Figure 1). Finally, recent analyses have demonstrated the incorporation of several host-cell encoded proteins into the mature viral particle [6].

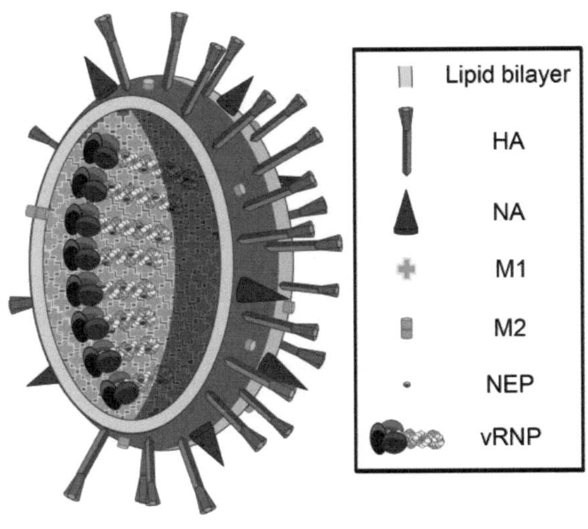

Figure 1.

1.2. A nuclear RNA virus: The life cycle of influenza A Virus

The infectious cycle of the virus starts with the binding of the infectious viral particle to the plasma membrane of the host cell. This initial binding is mediated by the viral HA protein, which exhibits high binding affinity for sialic acid molecules coating the extracellular domains of integral membrane proteins located at the plasma membrane. Upon binding, the virion enters the cell by receptor mediated endocytosis. Acidification of the resulting endocytic vesicle triggers the release of the vRNPs from the viral nucleocapsid and the fusion of the viral envelope with the endocytic membrane, thus allowing the discharge of the vRNPs into the cytoplasm of the infected cell [1]. Then, in a process mediated by cellular karyopherins, the vRNPs move rapidly into the nucleus (reviewed by Boulo et al. [7]). This nuclear translocation is a very peculiar and intriguing property of influenza virus, which makes it quite unique among RNA viruses, as most RNA viruses remain in the cytoplasm, where they carry out most of their functions, including viral replication. However, influenza virus requires access to the cell nucleus for successful transcription and replication of the viral genome. Once in the nucleus, the incoming RdRp associated to the vRNPs initiates synthesis of viral mRNA and produces the first round of viral protein synthesis, which leads to the expression of the early viral proteins PB1, PB2, PA, NP, and non-structural protein 1 (NS1) [1]. NS1, plays a critical role during infection by neutralizing cellular antiviral responses and increasing viral protein synthesis, while decreasing the synthesis of cellular proteins (reviewed by Hale et al. [8], Lin et al. [9], and Krug et al. [10]). The role of neutralizing antiviral defenses has been recently shown to be shared by another viral protein produced by a limited number of viral strains: The so-called PB1-F2 protein, a 90 amino acid protein produced by an alternative ORF contained within the PB1 gene segment [11-12].

Newly synthesized RdRps drive the synthesis of mRNA coding for late viral proteins, including HA, NA, M1, NS2, and M2, and later on undergo a shift in activity, from transcription to viral replication. Upon synthesis of new vRNA, the newly synthesized vRNA gene segments are incorporated into vRNPs that are exported out of the nucleus thanks to complex interactions established with the viral proteins NEP and M1, and the cellular karyopherin CRM1 [13]. The vRNPs are then incorporated into new viral particles by a budding process that takes place at lipid rafts located at the apical surface of the plasma membrane, in an area referred to as the budozone (reviewed by Vait and Thaa [14]). These lipid rafts contain the viral integral membrane proteins HA, NA, and M2, and the interactions established between the cytosolic tails of these proteins, particularly HA and NA, the viral structural protein M1, and vRNPs, appear to play a critical role as drivers of the budding process (reviewed by Nayak et al. [5], and Rossman and Lamb [3]). The budding process is completed by membrane scission, a process that involves the activity of M2 [15], and the infectious viral particles are released into the extracellular environment thanks to the activity of NA, which cleaves sialic acid molecules off the cell surface, therefore freeing the virus from interacting with its cellular receptor [3].

1.3. How influenza affects humans: Clinical effects of influenza in the human host

Seasonal epidemic influenza usually causes an acute but self-limited infection of the respiratory tract, characterized by acute febrile symptoms, sudden onset of sore throat, nonproductive cough, rhinorrhea, myalgia, headache, and general malaise. Uncomplicated influenza usually resolves within 3 to 7 days of the first appearance of symptoms, although the cough and the general malaise may persist for up to a couple of weeks [16]. Complicated influenza is usually associated to the presence of other pre-existing medical conditions in the infected person, including pulmonary or cardiac disease, diabetes, obesity, and hypertension. Complicated influenza may result in primary influenza viral pneumonia, lead to secondary bacterial pneumonia, or exacerbate other underlying medical conditions, most frequently of pulmonary or cardiac nature. Most of the complicated cases of influenza occur among people 65 years old and over. In the United States alone, seasonal epidemic influenza is estimated to be responsible for approximately 200,000 hospitalizations and 34,000 deaths every year [17-18]. Influenza has been shown to have strong pro-thrombotic and pro-inflammatory effects in the host. Therefore, a significant number of deaths associated with seasonal influenza infection are likely to be a consequence of cardiovascular events facilitated by pre-existing cardiovascular disease but triggered by influenza infection [19].

In contrast with the relative mildness of seasonal epidemic influenza, pandemic influenza usually has a more aggressive presentation. Pandemic influenza is associated with the introduction into the human host of a virus exhibiting an avian-type HA gene segment showing limited similarity to pre-existing human influenza viruses [20]. This determines that most humans will have few or no pre-existing cross-reactive antibodies against the avian-type HA protein that coats the viral particle, thus allowing unobstructed viral multiplication in the human host during the initial hours after infection. The fast viral growth that ensues under such conditions leads to a more aggressive disease presentation, accompanied sometimes by an unregulated cytokine production, a situation referred to as a "cytokine storm", that leads to an exaggerated pro-inflammatory response in the lungs [21]. Lung inflammation may in turn result in rapid progression to viral pneumonia, and in some cases to acute respiratory distress syndrome (ARDS), a condition that requires mechanical ventilation and may lead to death [20].

1.4. Our anti-influenza arsenal: Current therapeutic and prophylactic options against influenza

Currently, our most effective weapon against influenza virus is vaccination. However, effective vaccination requires a close antigenic match between the prevailing viral type being transmitted throughout the population and the viral strain used for vaccine development. The high mutational rate associated to the error prone viral RdRp, introduces frequent changes in the antigenic makeup of the virus. This imposes the need for an annual vaccination aimed at stimulating the immune system with a vaccine virus that closely resembles the changes occurring in the prevalent viral population. Selection of the viral strain to be used and vaccine production itself are both time consuming processes, and vaccine production against a novel pandemic virus may easily take 3 to 6 months, therefore keeping vaccination from playing an important role in the prevention of the first wave of viral infections during a pandemic, as recently evidenced during the 2009 H1N1 "swine" flu pandemic [22]. Further complicating the rapid production of anti-pandemic influenza vaccines is the potential undesired selection of viral variants that grow well in embryonated eggs, the current preferred media for amplification of the viral particles used for vaccine production. This may lead to the unintended selection of viral strains that are mismatched with the circulating viral strain [23].

A truly promising development related to influenza vaccines is the possibility of developing "universal" vaccines capable of triggering the production of broad-spectrum neutralizing antibodies effective against most (if not all) influenza strains. In addition to M2 and NP, the targets classically pursued for the development of universal influenza vaccines [24], it has been recently demonstrated the existence of two regions within the viral HA molecule that are capable of triggering broadly neutralizing antibodies: The stem and the receptor-binding pocket. Animal models have shown substantial progress in the ability to enhance the production of antibodies against the stem region, which is normally ignored by our immune system due to its inaccessibility [25]. However, it is still uncertain whether the success observed so far in animal models will be achievable in humans.

Antiviral drugs constitute our second most valuable weapon against influenza virus. Currently, there are two main types of FDA-approved anti-influenza drugs: Those targeting the viral M2 proton ion channel, which are chemically derived from Adamantane and therefore referred to as Adamantanes; and those targeting the viral neuraminidase protein, referred to as neuraminidase inhibitors. There are two M2 ion channel inhibitors: Amantadine (Symmetrel®) and Rimantadine (Flumadine®). These drugs act by blocking the ion channel formed by the M2 transmembrane protein, therefore preventing the acidification of the viral particle and precluding the release into the host cell cytoplasm of the vRNPs away from the viral matrix upon membrane fusion. Similarly, there are two neuraminidase inhibitors that are widely used in the clinic: Oseltamivir (Tamiflu®) and Zanamivir (Relenza®). These drugs act by inhibiting the enzymatic activity of the viral neuraminidase (NA) protein, therefore blocking viral release at the plasma membrane and preventing the spread of infection throughout the respiratory tract [26].

Although the two types of drugs indicated above have proven helpful at preventing and treating complicated cases of influenza, and as prophylactic tools to prevent influenza transmission among members of the same household, their clinical use has been limited by the viral ability to develop resistance against them. Resistance against the Adamantanes in tissue culture settings was rapidly noted after their initial development, but it was not recognized as a real issue until 2003 when widespread resistance to Adamantanes was first observed among clinical viral isolates in the USA. By 2005, resistance to Adamantanes was so predominant that their use was discontinued [27]. This situation did not change as a consequence of the 2009 pandemic, as the M2 gene segment in the 2009 H1N1 pandemic virus originated from an Adamantane resistant strain. Therefore, today virtually all circulating influenza strains in the USA are considered to be resistant to Adamantanes and their clinical use is no longer suggested by the CDC [28]. Resistance to Oseltamivir was initially considered to be much more difficult to develop and disseminate among circulating strains, mainly because the mutations involved in providing resistance to it were thought to reduce transmissibility and overall viral fitness [29]. However, over 99% of all clinical isolates of H1N1 influenza virus during the 2008-2009 influenza season were found to be resistant to Oseltamivir during the 2008-2009 influenza season [30-31]. Luckily, the NA gene incorporated into the H1N1 2009 pandemic virus was derived from an Oseltamivir-susceptible strain, and Oseltamivir resistance became substantially less predominant as the pandemic strain displaced and completely substituted the previous seasonal H1N1 strain. Nevertheless, resistance has already been reported among several clinical isolates of the currently circulating 2009 H1N1-derived influenza strain; therefore, it is likely that Oseltamivir resistance will become widespread among circulating viruses once again [32].

The vision that emerges from the brief review of our current anti-influenza arsenal presented above is one that emphasizes the need for alternative weapons. Vaccination will likely continue to play an essential role in minimizing the damaging effects of seasonal influenza, but unless we succeed in developing a truly universal anti-influenza vaccine, vaccination is unlikely to play a major role in the control of a highly pathogenic pandemic. Similarly, current antivirals may not be that useful either against a new pandemic due to the virus' ability to develop resistance against drugs targeting viral components. One promising alternative is to target cellular factors required for viral growth and multiplication for the development of new host-targeted antiviral agents [33-34]. One obvious drawback of this strategy is that drugs targeting host factors may exert toxic or substantial secondary effects in the host. However, host-targeted antiviral agents are likely to be effective against a broad range of viruses, (as most viral strains rely on the same cellular factors for their growth), and offer very limited chances for the development of viral resistance. In our opinion, these potential advantages associated to the implementation of host-targeted antivirals far outweigh their drawback and provide further justification for continuous investments aimed at a better understanding of influenza biology.

1.5. A hot affair that is about to happen emphasizes the need for further basic research: A highly pathogenic bird virus is likely to generate the next influenza pandemic

While many viruses are capable of producing severe disease in humans, few have the ability to generate pandemics with the potential to devastate human society. Influenza virus is one of them, and its ability to bring havoc into our society has been clearly demonstrated at least once in our recent historic record. The 1918 H1N1 "Spanish flu" influenza pandemic killed more than 50 million humans and probably infected over 30% of the human population at the time [35]. To date, the 1918 H1N1 pandemic is still considered the most damaging pandemic ever faced by humanity.

The isolation and characterization of the full array of viral gene segments of the 1918 pandemic virus, obtained from frozen and formalin-fixed tissue samples collected from victims of the 1918 pandemic, allowed the reconstruction of the virus [36]. This outstanding accomplishment has provided important insights into the molecular nature of the "Spanish flu" pandemic virus. Among others, those studies have revealed the relevance of specific gene segments, and of the full gene constellation as a whole, for the high pathogenicity exhibited by the virus (reviewed by Taubenberger and Kash [37]). However, numerous questions remain unsolved, including the origin of the virus. It has been postulated that the 1918 virus likely resulted from the direct adaptation of a bird virus to humans, based on molecular signatures of its genome, such as the high GC content [38]. However, others consider it more likely that the virus had been introduced initially into swine, therefore allowing it to gradually become adapted to mammals [39]. In the absence of a viral repository that could provide detailed knowledge of the predominant viral strains in the years before the 1918 pandemic, it is very likely that the actual origin of the 1918 pandemic will remain unknown.

The lack of evidence demonstrating that the 1918 pandemic virus jumped directly from birds into humans, the apparent adaptation of all subsequent pandemic viruses (including the recent 2009 H1N1 "swine flu" pandemic) in swine before their introduction in humans, and the notion that only three HA subtypes (H1, H2, and H3) are normally observed in humans, out of the sixteen different HA subtypes present in nature, helped maintain for decades the belief that avian influenza viruses could not be transmitted directly from birds to humans. This belief came to an end in May 1997 when a 3 year old boy in Hong Kong was infected and killed by what was subsequently determined to be an H5N1 avian virus [40-41]. Subsequent events of direct transmission of H5N1 avian viruses into humans have accounted for up to 597 human cases reported to the World Health Organization (WHO) as of 19 March 2012, 351 of which have been lethal, for a mortality rate of about 59% [42]. Furthermore, direct transmission from birds to humans has also been reported for H9N2 and H7N7 viral types[20].

It has been calculated that the mortality rate for the 1918 pandemic was approximately 2.5% [35]. Therefore, the apparent pathogenicity of H5N1 viruses for humans, suggested from the number of lethal cases, appears to surpass by a wide margin that of the 1918 "Spanish flu". However, the real mortality rate associated to H5N1 infections may be orders of magnitude lower, as suggested by numerous studies performed on the prevalence of antibodies against H5 (a measurement indicative of exposure to H5N1 viruses) among individuals in regions where clinical cases of H5N1 influenza have been reported [43]. Nevertheless, the high pathogenicity of the H5N1 virus for humans is unquestionable.

The factor that has precluded H5N1 from triggering a highly pathogenic human pandemic is its inability to be efficiently transmitted among humans. It has been almost 15 years since the first demonstrated case of direct transmission of H5N1 to humans, and throughout this time there has been arguably only one case of apparent direct H5N1 transmission among humans [44]. This suggests that it might be extremely difficult for the virus to become fully adapted for human transmission. Unfortunately, this may not be the case: Two recent reports, one published in Science by the group lead by Dr. Fouchier [45], and one published in Nature by the group lead by Dr. Kawaoka [46], and whose publication triggered substantial controversy due to the potential dual use of the data reported [47], provide proof that a few mutations affecting a limited number of viral gene segments are sufficient to allow highly pathogenic H5N1 viruses to become capable of direct transmission among ferrets, the animal model that best recapitulates the major features of influenza virus infections in humans . As the mutations identified in the Nature and Science reports could evolve spontaneously among viruses that propagate in the wild, these reports stress the relative high likelihood that humanity may face a highly pathogenic H5N1 pandemic sometime in the future. Importantly, other studies have also indicated that the novel 2009 H1N1 "swine flu" exhibits high genetic compatibility with highly pathogenic H5N1 viruses [48], thus also increasing the odds of H5N1 producing a human adapted high pathogenicity strain via reassortment with 2009 H1N1. Considering the weaknesses of our current anti-influenza defenses, these observations emphasize the utmost relevance of intensifying basic research in influenza biology with the goal of identifying and developing new prophylactic and therapeutic options against this virus.

2. Transcription and replication of the influenza virus genome

In the 1970's, Stephen C. Inglis, from the University of Cambridge at England, was the first to discover that the Influenza viral polymerase was a heterotrimeric protein complex composed of PB1, PB2, and PA. Later, further studies determined that NP, which encapsidates vRNA or complementary RNA (cRNA), forms large RNA-protein complexes when it associates with a viral polymerase and a cRNA or vRNA segment. In the past 40 years, the extensive characterization of each subunit of the viral polymerase, including NP, and the conserved sequences of the vRNA gene segments have provided substantial information contributing to our knowledge of the mechanisms employed by Influenza A virus for transcription and replication. However, despite the collective efforts of the influenza scientific community, some ambiguity still exists about how some steps take place during viral transcription and replication. In order to achieve a complete and detailed molecular knowledge of these processes, it is important to keep in perspective the basic knowledge previously established by the founders of the field and the most recent findings related to the regulation of the viral polymerase, all of which are briefly presented below.

2.1. The engine behind a pathogenic machinery: Nuclear accumulation and 3D structure of the viral RdRp

The release of the vRNPs from the infectious viral particle is perhaps the most critical step in the initiation of viral replication. This event requires the acidification of the viral particle core for the disruption of the intermolecular interactions shared between the vRNPs and the M1 viral protein [49]. The viral complex responsible for the acidification of the virion's core is the one formed by the tetramer of the M2 viral protein, which constitutes the smallest ion channel discovered to date [50]. The acidic environment then triggers the HA-mediated fusion of the viral and endosomal lipid bilayers [51-53], which allows the free vRNPs to migrate from the virion's core into the cytoplasm of the infected cell. Since influenza transcription and replication take place in the cell nucleus, the incoming vRNAs must then be imported into the nucleus, a process mediated by two nuclear localization signals (NLS) present in NP, (spanning residues 1-13 [NLS1] and residues 198-216 [NLS2]) [54]. Recent studies, performed using digitonin-permeabilized cells in the presence of exogenous cytosol and energy-regenerating systems, have suggested that the directionality of nuclear traffic of the vRNPs during infection is determined by the exposure or masking of NLS1 in NP [55]. However, even in the presence of an antibody against NLS1 in NP, vRNPs still migrate to the nucleoplasm, indicating that NLS2 in NP also contributes to the nuclear accumulation of vRNPs [54]. Additional studies are needed in order to assess the contribution of NLS2 in NP during the nuclear accumulation of the vRNPs.

The nuclear transport of the *de novo* synthesized viral polymerase proteins takes place in a highly organized manner and is critical for viral transcription and replication. The nuclear transport of PB2 occurs in the absence of any additional viral protein, while dimerization of PB1 and PA in the cytoplasm is required for their efficient nuclear trafficking [56-58]. Recent fluorescence cross-correlation spectroscopy (FCCS) studies demonstrated that the trimeric structure of the RdRp is only present inside the cell nucleus [57]. This finding led to the discovery of a new function for the N-terminal domain of PA; preventing the formation of these trimeric structures in the cytoplasm [59]. Unfortunately this inhibitory mechanism has not been fully characterized, but it is speculated that the flexible linker region separating the N- and C-terminal domains of PA allows for a conformational change that prevents binding of PB2 while residing in the cytoplasm. Should this be true, it would then be important to characterize the molecular mechanism triggering the conformational change in PA that takes place upon its entry in the nucleus.

The three subunits comprising the viral RNA-dependent RNA-polymerase (RdRp) are encoded by the three largest vRNA gene segments of Influenza A virus. PB2 is the largest subunit of the polymerase and the carrier of the 7-methylguanosine 5′-cap binding site [60]. The second largest subunit in the viral polymerase is PB1, and this is the only subunit that has the four conserved amino acids distributed among four different motifs present in all RNA-dependent RNA-polymerases and RNA-dependent DNA-polymerases [61]. Lastly, the smallest subunit, PA, has a characteristic PD-(D/E)-XK motif present in type II endonucleases, and is responsible for the cleavage of the 5′-cap of cellular mRNA [62-63]. These three viral factors form a very compact protein complex that still manages to maintain a high degree of flexibility.

Several different 3D conformations have been observed using cryo- and negative staining electron microscopy for the purified recombinant influenza viral polymerases in the presence or absence of vRNA, NP, and both [64-67]. Those studies demonstrated that the polymerase has a globular hollow conformation that becomes compacted upon association with vRNA alone or vRNA in the presence of NP oligomers [64-67]. Additionally, PB1, PB2, and NP have been identified as the main viral proteins mediating the RNA-dependent interaction of the viral polymerase and the RNA-protein complex formed between NP and vRNA [65]. The diverse array of quaternary structures portrayed by the molecular structures predicted for the viral polymerase in the studies mentioned above, provide strong evidence of the existence of multiple conformational stages for the polymerase, likely associated to its various functional properties during transcription and replication. However, multiple other structures such as those associated to the cRNA-bound stage, the 5′-cap interacting stage, and the oligomeric stage formed by the polymerase inside the nucleus, still remain unresolved.

2.2. Transcribing the blueprint to assemble the engine: Viral mRNA transcription

The transcription of the viral genome begins as early as one hour post-infection and takes place inside the cell nucleus [68] (Figure 2A). Early during infection, transcription of viral mRNAs is coupled to their translation and seems to plateau at 2.5 hours post-infection, whereas viral protein translation continues increasing throughout infection [68]. This provides evidence that a not fully characterized post-transcriptional regulatory mechanism ensures continued translation of the mRNA produced early during infection. Given that Influenza depends on the endogenous 5′ cap-dependent cellular ribosomal machinery to translate its gene products, influenza has developed a mechanism called "cap-snatching" to prime the synthesis of all viral mRNAs [69]. According to *in vitro* reconstitution assays the cap-snatching event seems to be dependent upon binding of the viral polymerase complex on the viral promoter at the 3′-end of vRNA molecules [63, 69-70]. This interaction between the viral RdRp and the 3′-end of the vRNA triggers a conformational change within the RdRp, and allows PB2 to bind the 7-methylguanosine 5′-cap from cellular mRNAs [60, 69]. Additionally, the interaction between the viral RdRp and the cellular mRNA brings into close proximity the cellular 5'-cap with the PD-(D/E)-XK motif in PA, which then enzymatically cleaves 9-17 nucleotides downstream of the 5′-cap at guanine or adenine residues [63, 71] (Figure 2B). Through the use of site directed mutagenesis, vRNP reconstitution assays, and primer extension analysis it has been further shown that the coordination of a divalent ion (preferably manganese or magnesium) by the N-terminal domain of PA is required for the cap-snatching event [62-63]. The divalent cation required for the endonucleolytic activity of PA is stabilized by a cluster of four residues (H41, E80, D108, E119) residing in the N-terminal domain of PA [62-63]. Moreover, the crystal structure of these four residues seems to be unusually distant from the catalytically active Lysine residue at position 134, when compared to other crystal structures of type II endonucleases [62-63]. As mentioned above, the 5′-cap from cellular mRNAs is used by the viral polymerase to prime the transcription of viral mRNA during infection [69, 72](Figure 2C). This phenomenon has been demonstrated by *in vitro* transcription assays in which the chemical removal of the 5′-cap from β-globin mRNA abolished the synthesis of viral mRNA [72]. Consistently, recapping of the β-globin mRNA through the use of a Vaccinia virus guanylyl or methyl transferase rescued the production of IAV mRNA [72].

While the 5′-cap from cellular mRNAs primes the transcription of viral mRNAs, the addition of ~150 adenines at the 3′ end, independent of the cellular poly-adenylation machinery, finalizes viral mRNA elongation. Polyadenylation of viral mRNAs is mediated by "stuttering" of the viral polymerase upon reaching a uridine-rich sequence usually made of 5-7 uridines, located 17 to 22 nucleotides away from the 5′ end of the vRNA template [73] (Figure 2D). At first, it was hypothesized that the formation of a panhandle structure between the complementary regions located at the 3′ and 5′ ends of the vRNA created sufficient steric hindrance to prevent the viral polymerase from transcribing the complete vRNA molecule, allowing the polyadenylation of viral mRNAs [73-74]. Later, *in vitro* transcription assays, performed using vRNA segments with various point mutations at the 5′-end as templates for transcription, determined that the formation of a duplex between the 3′- and 5′-ends of the vRNA, along with the binding of the viral polymerase to the 5′-end of the vRNA are both required for transcription [75]. This finding led to a refined hypothesis in which the viral polymerase binds to the panhandle structure formed between the complementary regions of the vRNA, recognizes the viral promoter, and subsequently elongates viral mRNA transcripts while remaining bound to the 5′-end of the template [75]. Because the viral polymerase is bound to the 5′-end of the template throughout the course of transcription, the viral polymerase is not capable of transcribing the 5′-end of the vRNA [75]. In other words, upon reaching the uridine-rich region at the 5′-end of the vRNA, the restraints inflicted by the intermolecular interactions shared between 5′-end of the vRNA and the viral polymerase will produce polymerase stuttering, and this in turn will allow polyadenylation to occur [75]. Subsequent studies proved that transcription of viral mRNA was mediated primarily by the incoming vRNP-bound polymerase and not by polymerases added in *trans* [76]. This unexpected but important data was obtained during vRNP transfection experiments in which the transcription of viral RNA introduced into the cell as a component of purified vRNPs formed in the presence of a mutated (transcriptionally inactive) PB2 subunit could not be rescued by the addition of recombinant functional polymerases [76]. Moreover, vRNP co-transfection experiments have shown that the transcription of viral gene segments could not take place by polymerases present on adjacent vRNPs [76]. Altogether, the results discussed above strongly suggest that transcription of viral mRNA is driven by the polymerases that accompany the vRNA into the nucleus in the form of vRNPs early during infection.

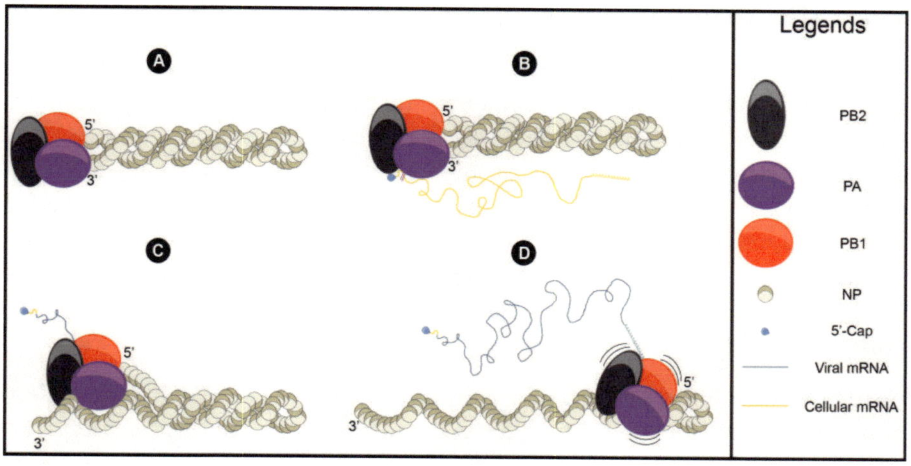

Figure 2.

2.3. The time and place to make the mistakes that might help future viral generations: Viral genome replication

The replication of the influenza virus genome requires the vRNA to first be transcribed into an additional type of viral RNA known as complementary RNA (cRNA). cRNA has a positive polarity and, as its name implies, it possesses a sequence that is complementary to that of the vRNA molecule. It is imperative for genome replication that the cRNA molecule contains the complete sequence of the vRNA, since it will be used as the template that will drive the synthesis of new vRNA late during infection. Early studies demonstrated that, in sharp contrast with the transcription of mRNA, the transcription of cRNA can be initiated in a primer-independent manner, while also using the same 13 and 12 nucleotides at the 5′- and 3′-end of the vRNA respectively as a promoter for transcription [77-78]. However, despite cRNA molecules being used for the replication of the viral genome, the accumulation of cRNA is very limited at early time points during infection [77]. It was also shown that the transcription of complete vRNA segments from cRNA templates could not be achieved in the absence of NP during *in vitro* transcription assays [79]. Subsequently, it was demonstrated that the absence of cRNA at early time points post-infection could be explained by the lack of free NP protein early during infection, because the artificially driven expression of NP within the cell before infection allowed the accumulation of cRNA at early time points post-infection [80]. The model developed based on these observations proposed the formation of a "stabilization complex", in which the binding and coating of the cRNA molecule with NP monomers prevents its degradation by cellular RNAses [80]. Surprisingly, even after 30 years of research, not very much information has been gathered on the molecular mechanisms involved in the elongation of cRNAs or how the steric hindrances faced by the viral polymerase during transcription are evaded to permit the complete transcription of the cRNA segment.

2.4. Knowing when to stop and accelerate leads to a more pathogenic performance: Mechanisms regulating transcription and replication

The meticulous orchestration of the multiple molecular complexes formed between the viral polymerase, vRNA, cRNA, other viral proteins, and cellular factors throughout the various steps during viral transcription and replication, provides additional molecular targets and mechanisms to regulate the activity of the RdRp. Those interactions are constantly triggering conformational changes on the flexible structure of the viral polymerase, which in turn dictate the specific functionality that it should exert. In order to further exemplify how different molecular interactions can exert a regulatory function on the viral polymerase, the structure of the viral promoter and the role of other viral proteins interacting with the RdRp will be discussed briefly below.

i) The structure of the viral promoters: Through the use of Nuclear Magnetic Resonance (NMR) and calculations for determining the 3D structure of the vRNA promoter, it has been shown that the vRNA promoter has a terminal stem, followed by an internal loop, and a proximal stem [81-82]. The terminal stem displays an inherent bend that allows the viral promoter to be easily melted, therefore possibly playing a regulatory role during the initiation of RNA synthesis [82]. This intrinsic bending of the terminal stem might be of great relevance for transcription initiation, since the viral RdRp does not appear to have a helicase activity associated to it [82]. Additionally, the nucleotides involved in the formation of the internal loop within the vRNA promoter correspond to the same nucleotides previously identified as the binding sites for the viral RdRp [82-83]. Most of the residues constituting the internal loop have a highly dynamic structure and their binding to the viral polymerase creates an energetically favorable reaction by reducing the high entropy displayed by this structure [82]. Therefore, it is suggested that this internal loop in the vRNA promoter positions the catalytic core of the viral polymerase at the transcription initiation site [82].

The structure of the cRNA promoter used for genome replication has also been determined by NMR and exhibits a somewhat comparable but very distinct structure to that of the vRNA promoter [84]. Importantly, the structural differences between the two viral promoters might allow the viral polymerase to distinguish between the transcription of mRNA/cRNA and vRNA [84]. This idea is further supported by the fact that the viral polymerase binds to the cRNA promoter through the central region of PB1, while the vRNA promoter interacts with the C-terminal region of PB1 [85]. Interestingly, in both cases the internal loop regions of the vRNA and cRNA are involved in the binding of the RdRp, suggesting that the structure of the internal loop might be more relevant than the actual sequence itself for positioning the viral polymerase to initiate transcription [84-85]. Nonetheless, even though the internal loop regions share general structural similarities, their individual conformations are quite distinct. The comparison of both structures showed that the internal loop of the cRNA promoter is very unstable when compared to the internal loop present in the vRNA promoter [84]. The lack of stability of the internal loop region in the cRNA is due to the improper stacking of the bases belonging to the nucleotides located in that region, which contrasts sharply with the proper stacking observed for the nucleotides located in the equivalent regions of the vRNA promoter [84]. However, the relevance of such great difference in stability for both the vRNA and cRNA loop regions still remains unknown.

ii) Viral proteins involved in the regulation of the viral polymerase: As mentioned above, viral proteins different from those constituting the vRNP complexes can also play an important regulatory role in the function of the viral polymerase. To date, the molecular mechanisms underlying the viral polymerase switch from transcription to replication still remain unresolved. However, the involvement of several viral factors has been characterized to some degree. So far, only one viral protein has been identified as a regulator of the transcriptase activity of the viral polymerase. Primer extension analyses, have shown that the mRNA/vRNA ratio generated during vRNP reconstitution assays performed in the presence of NP and the viral RdRp (but no other viral protein) is substantially larger than the mRNA/vRNA ratio normally generated during viral infection [86]. Testing the effect of overexpressing individual Influenza A viral proteins on the transcription of multiple vRNA gene segments during vRNP reconstitution assays allowed the identification of a transcriptional regulatory function associated with NEP [86]. Subsequently, it was shown that the presence of NEP leads to the generation of Influenza A virus-derived small viral RNAs (svRNA) [87]. These svRNAs correspond to the 5′-end of each vRNA genomic segment and have different lengths, ranging from 22 to 27 nucleotides, depending on the gene segment they are derived from, and seem to interact directly with the viral polymerase [87]. More importantly, their accumulation in the cell is coupled to a shift from viral transcription to replication, while their depletion results in loss of vRNA synthesis for their parental gene segment [87]. These results suggest that these svRNAs prime the initiation of transcription for genomic vRNA, as previously observed in cellular DNA-dependent RNA-polymerases. Altogether, both NEP and svRNAs seem to be playing a critical role in the switch from transcription to replication. Nevertheless, no direct interaction between the polymerase and NEP has been observed through the use of immunoprecipitation assays, therefore leaving the exact molecular mechanism involved in this regulatory process unresolved. An important lesson derived from these studies is that, in the absence of supplementary proteins (e.g. NEP) the limited number of viral factors (PB1, PB2, PA, and NP), commonly employed during vRNP reconstitution assays, might prevent us from realizing the authentic effects imposed by chemical inhibitors or point mutations on the transcriptase activity of the RdRp, since under such conditions these assays do not accurately recapitulate the events involved in viral transcription and replication during influenza infections.

3. Cellular factors important for viral multiplication

The first identification of cellular factors involved in influenza viral infection took place as early as 1959 [88]. However, up to fairly recent times, most studies related to influenza replication and multiplication focused exclusively on the mechanistic assessment of processes mediated by viral proteins and put little emphasis on the cellular factors or pathways involved in influenza replication. During the last few years, the use of multiple approaches such as protein pull-downs, chemical inhibition studies, yeast-two hybrid screening, affinity purification, and RNA interference (RNAi), have led to the identification of multiple cellular factors essential for influenza viral replication [89-97]. In the sections below, we will review the most recent findings related to the relevance of specific host cellular proteins and systems for influenza transcription and replication. Despite the substantial progress achieved during the last few years, the overall status quo of the field is that the functions of the characterized viral-cellular protein interactions remain mostly unclear. Table 1 summarizes the cellular factors required for influenza replication discussed in this section.

3.1. Downloading a virus: Viral egress from endocytic vesicles

In order for the vRNPs to reach the nucleus, which constitutes their final destination within the host cell, they have to be released from the incoming viral particle. This process requires the acidification of the viral particle and fusion of the endosomal and viral membranes. The decrease in pH within the endosomal compartment requires the cellular vacuolar proton ATPases (v-(H^+)ATPase) to hydrolyze ATP and transport protons inside the vesicle [98]. Three large screenings for cellular factors relevant for influenza infection, performed by Hao et al. [91], Konig et al. [92], and Karlas et al. [95], identified members of the v-(H^+)ATPase family as critical host factors required for the progression of influenza infection. Before the screenings, it had been established that treatment of cells with concanamycin A, a well known inhibitor of v-(H^+)ATPases, was enough to halt the production of viral proteins at an early stage post-infection. However, the addition of concanamycin A one hour after infection had no effect on the production of viral proteins, suggesting that the inhibition of endosome acidification affected only the earliest stages of viral infection [99]. Subsequent studies using diverse inhibitors and RNAi approaches confirmed the involvement of v-(H^+)ATPases in early stages of infection [100-101] and provided further details of their specific role during influenza infections [102]. Studies by Marjuki et al. [102] revealed that, upon entering the cell, influenza activates the ERK and PI3K pathways. These pathways activate the E subunit of the v-(H^+)ATPase V1 domain, upregulating its proton pumping activity and leading to a more rapid acidification of the endosome [102], a process needed for the fusion of the viral and endosomal membranes.

The non-clathrin-coated vesicular coat COP-I proteins have also been identified as important cellular factors required for efficient viral replication in three large viral-cellular interaction screenings (Table 1.), thus supporting a relevant role for this protein family in the influenza life cycle. However, it is still uncertain the specific events in the viral life cycle that are affected by this protein family. Because one of the screenings that identified the COP-I proteins as relevant for viral infection used the transcription of early viral genes as output, and the known role of COP-I proteins in retrograde traffic of Golgi vesicles back to the ER [103], it is likely that the COP-I proteins are necessary for some stage of viral entry.

Onward from endocytosis of the viral particles, it has been suggested that a member of the lysosome-associated membrane glycoprotein family, LAMP3, is involved in the release of the vRNPs from the endosomal compartments and in facilitating vRNP nuclear import. However, the hypothetical pivotal role suggested for LAMP3 during infection is somewhat surprising, since LAMP3 is interferon induced and up-regulated during viral infection and therefore expected to exert an anti-viral activity. Nevertheless, siRNA knockdown of LAMP3 significantly reduced levels of NP expression during infection [104], thus supporting the enhancing role postulated for LAMP3.

3.2. A molecular hijacker: Nuclear shuttling of vRNPs

Once inside the cytoplasm, viral RNA transcription begins only upon arrival of the viral ribonucleoprotein (vRNP) complexes into the nucleus. The shuttling across the nuclear pore complex of both, the largest macromolecular complexes formed by the virus during infection, i.e. the vRNPs, as well as of its individual protein components, rely on the cellular nucleocytoplasmic trafficking machinery. The importin α/β pathway is the classical nuclear import pathway, transporting cargo proteins from the cytoplasm into the nucleus upon recognition of a nuclear localization sequence (NLS) by karyopherins, typically importin α. Most cargo proteins directly interact through their NLS with the adapter protein importin α, which then binds importin β for nuclear import. Transport of the importin α/β-cargo protein complex is facilitated by interactions with nucleoporins (Nups), the structural components of the nuclear pore complex [105]. Expectedly, Nups were one the major categories of factors identified in large scale screenings for cellular proteins required for efficient influenza infections, having been identified in 4 different screenings [92-93, 95, 97]. Their fundamental role as regulators of nucleocytoplasmic traffic allows them to dictate the nucleocytoplasmic transport of viral transcripts, proteins, and RNPs.

The PB2 and NP viral proteins have been shown to interact with importin $\alpha 1$ for their nuclear trafficking. As previously described, NP contains two NLS, both of which are of great relevance for proper nuclear import of vRNPs, since mutating either of the two NLS domains results in decreased accumulation of vRNPs within the nucleus [54]. As for PB2, its interaction with importin $\alpha 1$ was initially characterized through targeted mutations in the aspartic acid at position 701 and asparagine at position 319. These two point mutations on PB2 have the ability to further enhance its affinity for importin $\alpha 1$, and consequently, its nuclear accumulation [106]. Furthermore, studies using Fluorescence Cross-Correlation Spectroscopy (FCCS), in which the live transient trafficking of transiently expressed viral

Reference	Mayer et al. (43)	Jorba et al. (48)	Hao et al. (47)	Konig et al. (46)	Brass et al. (45)	Shapira et al. (44)	Karlas et al. (42)	Bortz el al. (10)	Tafforeau et al. (11)	Literature Based
Cellular Interactors Identified by	RdRp purification (PB1/ PB2/ PA)	RdRp purification (PB1/ PB2/ PA)	RNAi Approach	RNAi Approach	RNAi Approach	Yeast Two-Hybrid	RNAi Approach	RNAi Approach	Yeast Two-Hybrid with vRdRp (PB1/PB2/PA)	Host Factors Discussed, Not Present in Screens
Endocytic vRNP Release			ATPVOD1	ATP6AP1, ATP6AP2, ATP6V1A, ATP6V1B2, ATP6VOB, ATP6VOC, ATP6VOD1			ATP1A2, ATP6AP1, ATP6AP2, ATP2C1, ATP6VOC, ATP6VOD1, ATP6V1A, ATPV1B2			LAMP3
Nuclear Import	KPNA1, KPNA2, KPNB3				KPNA1, KPNAB1, RAN	KPNA1, KPNA3, KPNA6	KPNB1	KPNA1, KPNA4, KPNB3		
Transcription and Replication	POLII(CTD)	SFPQ/PSF		EIF2AK2	POLRH2, EIF2S1		POLRH2, POLR2L, EIF4A3, EIF3A, EIF3C, EIF3G	SFPQ	POLR2A, EIF3S6IP	TFIIH, P-TEFb, PSF
vRNA Splicing	UAP56						CLK1			SF2/ASF
Nuclear export and Membrane Migration			NXF1	PRKC1, MAPEK/MEK, MAPK1/ERK, RAB11, RAB17, RABEP1, NUP214, NUP153, NTRK2	NXF1, NUP62, NUP88, NUP98, NUP107, NUP214, NUPL1	RABGEF1	NXF1 XPO1(CRM1), RAB6B, NUP98, NUP205,		NUP54	URH49, REF/ALY, RAF/MEK/ERK, PDGFR, PABP1, FPPS, CDK1, CDK2, CDK5
Apoptosis	HSP90			HSP90, PRKC1, PRKCD, PRKACA, PRKAG2			HSP90			
Other Viral-Host Pathways	PARP1			SUMO1, SUMO2, SUMO4, SAE1, ARCN1 (COPD), COPA, COPB, COPG	ARCN1 (COPD), COPA, COPB1, COPG, COPZ1, COPS6	SUMO1P1, UBE21	UBAC2, COPA, COPB1, COPB2, COPG,	PARP1	COPS5	ERK, PI3K

Table 1. Summarized Host Factors Involved in Influenza Replication and Viral Processes.

proteins is recorded, confirmed the interaction between PB2 and importin α during its nuclear import. In contrast with the use of the classical nuclear traffic pathway by PB2, the FCCS studies also noted that nuclear traffic of the remaining viral polymerase subunits (PB1 and PA) occurs through a non-conventional importin α-independent pathway [57], with PB1 forming a heterodimer with PA, which is required by PB1 and PA to gain access to the nucleus (as stated in section 4a) and using it in conjunction with Ran binding protein 5 (RanBP5) as the carrier [107].

3.3. Someone's in the kitchen: Cellular dependent transcription and vRNA synthesis

The activation of RdRp driven vRNA transcription relies heavily on the host cell transcriptional machinery. Four different viral-host interaction screenings [89, 93, 95, 97] identified subunits of the cellular RNA Polymerase II (Pol II), which further reinforced previous work performed on the proposed mechanisms for the role of Pol II on viral transcription. During the normal cycle of cellular RNA transcription, the promoter associated Pol II is phosphorylated by TFIIH to initiate transcription. Transcription, however, can be temporarily paused by negative elongation factors, allowing time for the addition of the 5′ cap to the short segment of pre-mRNA transcript already synthesized. Subsequent phosphorylation of the C-terminal domain of the paused Pol II, mediated by P-TEFb, relieves the pause and re-activates transcription [108]. Before the onset of viral transcription, the viral PB2 protein, in association with PB1 and PA, is brought into close proximity to the cellular Pol II by TFIIH, allowing it to bind the 5′-cap structure of a cellular pre-mRNA transcript [109]. As described in the previous section, PA steals the 5′-cap along with a 9-17 nucleotide extension in a mechanism referred to as "cap-snatching." The 5′-cap oligonucleotide then serves as a primer for the polymerase subunit of the RdRp, PB1, to initiate vRNA transcription and elongation [110]. Elongation ends when the RdRp reaches a 5 to 7 uridine base-pair extension towards the 5′ end of the vRNA template, which signals for polyadenylation of the transcript [111-112]. Cell splicing factors also appear to be vital for efficient vRdRp-dependent transcription of the viral genome. In a reporter assay, knockdown of the nuclear Splicing Factor Proline-Glutamine Rich (SFPQ/PSF) reduced levels of viral transcription, but had no effect on viral genome replication. Moreover, *in vitro* analysis of viral transcription revealed about a ~5-fold reduction in the fraction of viral polyadenylated (positive sense) transcripts, suggesting that SFPQ/PSF seems to facilitate the polyadenylation of viral transcripts [113]. UAP56, (Bat1/Raf-2p48), a known viral-interactor protein that was also identified in a vRdRp interaction screening by Mayer et al. [89], is a fairly well established RNA helicase involved in spliceosome assembly [114], facilitating the nuclear export of cellular mRNA [115], and is a constituent of the transcription export complex which delivers pre-mRNAs bound to the exon-junction complex to nuclear export factor 1 (NXF1) [116]. Although UAP56 is clearly a factor in cellular RNA splicing, *in vitro* studies indicate that UAP56 forms heterodimers with NP in the absence of vRNA. Upon addition of vRNA the heterodimer dissociates and, through an unknown mechanism, facilitates vRNA synthesis [117] suggesting higher affinity interaction of one of these proteins for vRNA. Altogether, this not only suggests a pro-viral functionality of UAP56 in enhancing vRNA production, but that efficient viral replication exploits multiple functionalities of cellular host factors in a well orchestrated manner.

3.4. Cutting and mincing the viral transcripts: Host splicing machinery and influenza viral RNA

Splicing of viral mRNA, needed for the production of M2 and NS2, is fully dependent on the host splicing machinery due to the lack of splicing factors encoded within the viral genome. However, the splicing of the M viral segment to produce the M2 transcript is orchestrated by both viral and cellular components. CDC-like kinase 1 (CLK1), a protein responsible for the regulation of pre-mRNA splicing, plays a key role in the production of M2 vRNA spliced transcripts as demonstrated through RNAi knock-down and chemical inhibition studies [95]. CLK1 has been implicated in regulating the splicing of M1 mRNA [95], by phosphorylating the serine/arginine rich splicing factor, SF2/ASF [118]. SF2/ASF is a member of the serine/arginine rich splicing factor family, which are key factors in both alternative and constitutive pre-mRNA splicing, (reviewed in [119]) and is a critical splicing factor involved in the production of M2. Although cellular transcripts most often rely on consistent excision of intronic sequences, influenza virus replication depends on precise proportions of spliced and unspliced transcripts, as observed in the processing of the M1 mRNA transcript. For the duration of infection, splicing factor SF2/ASF is associated to a purine-rich enhancer sequence on the 3′ end exon of the M1 transcript. In early stages of infection, the 5′ $mRNA_3$ splicing donor site of the M1 RNA transcript is the highly preferred splicing donor site by the host splicing machinery, thus causing the disfavored M2 5′ splicing donor site, ~40 nucleotides downstream, to be ignored. As infection progresses, a newly synthesized viral RdRp binds the 5′ end of the unspliced M1 mRNA, blocking access of the cellular splicing machinery to the $mRNA_3$ 5′ end splice donor site. [120]. The host splicing machinery then associates with the M2 5′ splice donor site, awaiting activation by SF2/ASF to initiate production of M2 mRNA transcripts [121]. Host splicing factors involved in the processing of the eighth gene segment, NS segment, have yet to be specified. Although it appears that the competition between the splicing machinery and the nucleocytoplasmic transport machinery regulate the production of NEP, it has been established that viral factors associated with viral infection do not regulate splicing of the NS transcript [122-123].

3.5. Unexpected delivery: Nuclear export of Viral mRNA and the vRNP

Since IAV has the unique capability among RNA viruses of replicating in the nucleus, there are additional processes such as viral mRNA and vRNP nuclear export that are essential for viral infection. Due to the nature of the "cap-snatching" event that takes place during infection, nuclear cap-binding complexes have the ability to interact with viral mRNAs and aid in the recruitment of nuclear export regulatory factors such as REF/Aly [124]. This was shown through the use of simple interaction studies in which viral mRNA was able to co-immunoprecipitate with translational machinery factors such as cellular cap binding proteins, RNA and export factor-binding protein REF/Aly, cellular poly(A)-binding protein 1 (PABP1), the 20 kDa subunit of the nuclear cap-binding complex (NCBP2), and the eukaryotic translation initiation factor 4E (eIF4E) [124]. Additional cellular factors involved in viral mRNA nuclear export were also identified by multiple RNAi screenings. These studies revealed that independent viral mRNA transcripts exploit specific nuclear export factors for their individual export into the cytoplasm. It was not surprising that NXF1, a cellular protein involved in the nuclear export of cellular mRNAs, was found to be of relevance for influenza replication in three independent screenings [91, 93-95]. siRNA knockdowns against NXF1 revealed that mRNAs coding for the early protein NS1, and the late proteins HA, NA, M1, and M2, depend on NXF1 for their nuclear export [91, 93-95]. The mRNAs encoding for the viral polymerase proteins PB1, PB2, PA, and NP also show dependence on NXF1 for their nuclear export, but to a lesser extent [125]. On the other hand, the nuclear export of mRNAs coding for M1, M2, and NS1 show dependence on the previously mentioned RNA helicase, UAP56, for their efficient nuclear export [126]. The dependence of these transcripts on UAP56 was demonstrated by knocking down UAP56, or its high sequence identity paralog URH49. The limited availability of either UAP56 or URH49 triggered an accumulation of influenza dsRNA at the nuclear membrane and an increase in IFN production [126]. However, even when the multiple RNAi screenings have identified cellular factors like NXF1 and UAP56 as essential for viral mRNA nuclear export, additional factors such as those involved in the nuclear export of the mRNA for NEP still remain unknown. Also, we still need to identify the other proteins forming the complexes involved in nuclear export of viral mRNAs, to facilitate the complete characterization of the molecular mechanism driving this fundamental process.

As mentioned above, vRNP nuclear export is also a process of great relevance for the assembly of infectious viral particles. So far, we know that mature vRNP complexes depend on the CRM1 pathway for their nuclear export. CRM1 mediated nuclear export is carried out through the recognition of a nuclear export signal (NES) present in the amino acid sequence of the cargo protein [127]. In the case of the vRNPs, CRM1 binds to the NES located at the N-terminal region of NEP. Interestingly, after mutating the NES present in NEP, its nuclear export was impaired without affecting its interaction with CRM1 [13]. Crystallographic studies of the M1 binding domain present in NEP suggested that the nuclear export of vRNPs required the formation of a "daisy-chain complex" in which, RanGTP-loaded CRM1 associates with the N-terminal NES of NEP, and NEP is associated via its C-terminal domain to an M1 molecule bound C-terminally to the vRNP [128]. Furthermore, several studies have identified a structural component of the nuclear pore complex involved in CRM1-dependent export, Nucleoporin 98 (Nup98), as a critical host factor during influenza A viral replication [91, 93, 95, 129]. A recent study demonstrated the interaction between a GLFG repeat domain located within the Nup98 protein and NEP [129]. This interaction suggests that Nup98 facilitates nuclear export of the vRNPs during influenza infection, via its interaction with NEP [129]. To confirm the relevance of the GLFG domain in Nup98 during viral infection, a mutant form of Nup98 lacking the GLFG domain was overexpressed by transfection and led to a substantial decrease in viral titers [129]. Even though the studies described above provide evidence that Nup98 is an essential cellular factor for viral infection, a more detailed knowledge of the molecular events mediating vRNP nuclear export is still missing.

Lastly, after leaving the nucleus, the vRNPs need to migrate towards the apical surface of the cell to become encapsidated into new virions. Previous studies demonstrated through the use of live imaging microscopy that, upon entering the cytoplasm, vRNP complexes associate with a pericentriolar recycling endosome marker called Rab11, which is involved in endosomal recycling and trafficking [130]. The accumulation of vRNPs at the microtubule-organizing center after nuclear export, allows them to interact with Rab11-positive recycling endosomes and migrate along microtubules to the sites of budding at the apical surface of the plasma membrane [131-133].

4. Influenza virus and the cellular SUMOylation system

4.1. A cellular system with a funny name: Generalities of the SUMOylation system

SUMOylation, the post-translational conjugation of the Small Ubiquitin-like MOdifier (SUMO) to a protein, involves the formation of an isopeptide link between the carboxyl group located at the C-terminal glycine residue in SUMO and the epsilon amino group in a lysine residue located internally in the target protein. There are four different SUMO molecules in humans, SUMO 1-4. SUMO2 and SUMO3 are 95% identical to each other, and in consequence are usually referred to simply as SUMO2/3, whereas SUMO1 shares only approximately 50% identify with them (reviewed by Geiss-Friedlander and Melchior [134], and Dohmen [135]). Besides their sequence differences, SUMO2/3 and SUMO1 appear to be functionally different as well: First, the pool of proteins that are SUMOylated with SUMO2/3 is only partially overlapping with the pool of proteins that are SUMOylated with SUMO1 [136-137]; second, SUMO2/3 is capable of forming poly-SUMO2/3 chains in vivo, whereas SUMO1 is not (reviewed by Ulrich [138]). The ability of SUMO4 to be conjugated to proteins *in vivo* is still being debated and therefore its biological role is still uncertain.

The enzymatic pathway involved in SUMOylation resembles that required for the conjugation of its related protein, Ubiquitin, and consists of an E1 activating and an E2 conjugating enzymes, a set of E3 ligases, and a set of SUMO-specific peptidases and isopeptidases (Figure 3). However, the specific enzymes required for SUMOylation are distinct from those involved in Ubiquitinylation, and therefore the Ubiquitin and SUMO pathways are independent from each other and subject to different regulatory mechanisms. Interestingly, while in the Ubiquitin pathway the conjugation of Ubiquitin to a substrate has an absolute requirement for the involvement of an E3 Ubiquitin ligase, in the SUMO pathway the E1 and E2 activities (performed by the heterodimeric protein SAE2/SAE1 and Ubc9, respectively) are sufficient for SUMO conjugation, without the absolute need for an E3 SUMO ligase. Nevertheless, numerous E3 SUMO ligases have been identified and are considered to play an important regulatory role for the SUMOylation of specific targets in vivo (reviewed by Dohmen [135], Geiss-Friedlander and Melchior [134], and Wilson and Heaton [139]). The SUMO peptidases and isopeptidases make SUMOylation a reversible modification, and their high intracellular concentration and activity is thought to be responsible for the low cellular concentration of the SUMOylated form for any given protein (for most SUMO targets, the SUMOylated form of the target represents less than 5% of the steady-state cellular level of that protein) [140].

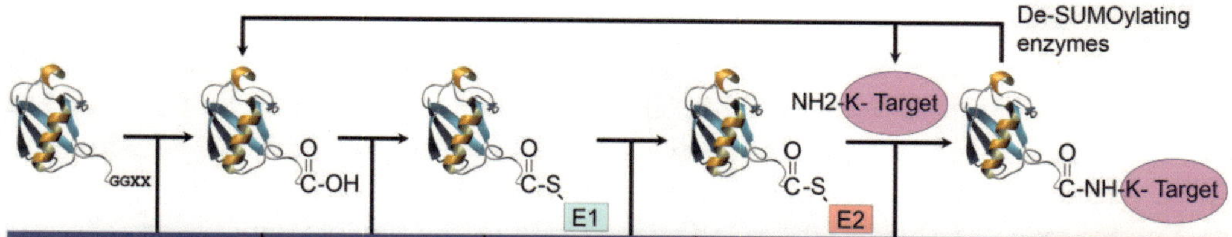

Maturation and De-SUMOylation	E1-activating enzymes	E2-conjugating enzyme	E3-ligases	Enzymatic step
Six known enzymatically active sentrin-SUMO specific proteases in humans (SENP1, 2, 3, 5, 6, 7) and an additional enzyme DeSUMOylating isopeptidase-1 (DeSI-1)	A single heterodimeric E1-activating enzyme (SAE1/SAE2; AOS1/UBA2)	Single E2-conjugating enzyme (Ubc9; Ube2I)	Ten known ligases grouped into three groups: proteins containing SP-RING domains (PIAS proteins), proteins lacking RING domains (RanBP2 and Pc2), and TOPORS (topoisomerase 1-binding, arginine/serine-rich)	Characteristics

Figure 3.

4.2. A "molecular matchmaker": The effects of SUMOylation on its target proteins

SUMOylation is known to affect an ever increasing number of cellular proteins, some of which were initially identified as SUMO targets during large-scale proteomic analyses of cellular SUMOylation [136-137, 141-142]. The effects produced by this post-translational modification on its target proteins are numerous and appear to be protein specific. Among others, SUMO has been shown to alter its target proteins by affecting their cellular localization, protein stability/half-life, and protein activity (reviewed by Hay [140], Hilgart et al. [143], Gill [144], and Wilkinson and Henley [145]). The unifying theme behind the wide range of activities mediated by SUMOylation appears to be SUMO's ability to regulate the intermolecular interactions established between its targets and other macromolecules, sometimes enhancing them and sometimes blocking them. In either case, it seems that whatever the effect mediated by SUMO might be, its effects last longer than the actual SUMOylated state of the target. In other words, the protein interactions facilitated or prevented by SUMOylation are maintained even after the protein has been de-SUMOylated. A simple explanation for this fact is that SUMO may act as a "molecular matchmaker", introducing proteins to each other and allowing them to establish long-lasting interactions, probably stabilized by the recruitment of other protein partners that can only interact with the interacting pair but not with the individual members of the pair. Those long-lasting interactions remain even after a de-SUMOylating enzyme takes away the SUMO molecule that allowed the initial interaction. As a consequence, mutations affecting the ability of a protein to become SUMOylated will have dramatic effects on protein function, despite the fact that the SUMOylated form of the protein may represent only a small fraction of its total in the cell.

4.3. A post-translational modification known to wrestle with many infectious organisms: The interplay between the cellular SUMOylation system and various infectious agents

While numerous infectious organisms are now known to interact with the cellular SUMOylation system by having some of their proteins being modified by SUMOylation, there are a few specific examples of infectious organisms that produce global changes in the activity of the cellular SUMOylation system. Interestingly, for such organisms capable of affecting the overall activity of the SUMOylation system, the predominant picture observed is their tendency to decrease both, the activity of the SUMOylation system and the overall number of SUMOylated proteins present within the host [146]. This trend suggests that the SUMOylation system may have an intrinsic effect as a cellular defense mechanism against some infectious agents. Two well characterized proteins encoded by two different infectious organisms, a virus and a bacterium, exemplify and support the predominant picture indicated above and, therefore, will be briefly discussed below.

i) Gam1: Gam1 is a protein encoded by the so-called chicken embryo lethal orphan (CELO) avian adenovirus. This protein was initially characterized as an anti-apoptotic viral protein, as well as an inhibitor of the deacetylating enzyme HDAC1 [147]. Subsequently, it was observed that Gam1 was also capable of inducing both, the loss of Pro-Myelocytic Leukemia Nuclear Bodies (PML-NBs), a nuclear structure believed to play antiviral activities and whose formation depends on the SUMOylation of the PML protein, and a global decrease in host cellular SUMOylation [148]. Follow up studies demonstrated that Gam1 inactivates the heterodimeric SUMO activating enzyme SAE2/SAE1, therefore triggering its degradation by a proteasomal-dependent pathway. The degradation of the E1 activating enzyme for the SUMO pathway also leads to the degradation of the E2 conjugating enzyme, Ubc9, therefore producing a complete block in SUMOylation [149]. Importantly, Gam1 has been demonstrated to be essential for CELO viral growth and multiplication, therefore suggesting that the SUMO inhibitory activity mediated by Gam1 is essential for viral fitness [150].

ii) Listeriolysin O (LLO): LLO is a pore forming toxin produced by the intracellular bacterial pathogen *Listeria monocytogenes*, the causative agent of human listeriosis. In a study aimed at evaluating the potential ability of *L. monocytogenes* to alter global cellular SUMOylation, it was observed that HeLa cells infected with this bacterium exhibited a dramatic decrease in global cellular SUMOylation. This was not true for HeLa cells infected with its non-pathogenic cousin *L. innocua*. Subsequent analysis of various bacterial mutants identified LLO as the factor responsible for the de-SUMOylating activity associated to *L. monocytogenes*. Specifically, LLO was shown to trigger the degradation of the E2 conjugating enzyme Ubc9, therefore leading to a global decrease in cellular SUMOylation. The relevance of this decrease for bacterial infection was demonstrated by showing that over-expression of SUMO1 or SUMO2 in HeLa cells before *L. monocytogenes* infection led to a substantial decrease in the number of intracellular bacteria produced by 7 h post-infection, thus supporting a role for decreased cellular SUMOylation in enhancing bacterial growth [151].

In contrast with the examples presented above, there are also reports of proteins encoded by viral pathogens that are endowed with the ability to enhance the SUMOylation of specific cellular proteins as a way to regulate cellular systems that play an important role during viral infection. Two important examples of this type of interaction between viral agents and the SUMOylation system are presented below.

iii) K-bZIP: The basic leucine zipper protein of Kaposi's sarcoma-associated herpesvirus (KSHV), K-bZIP, is one of the earliest proteins expressed after acute infection or reactivation by KSHV. K-bZIP, a transcriptional regulator of viral gene expression, was initially shown to interact with the SUMOylation system by acting as a SUMO target, being SUMOylated at residue K158. K-bZIP SUMOylation appeared to affect its transcriptional activity [152]. Subsequently, it was shown that K-bZIP contains a SUMO2/3-specific SUMO Interacting Motif (SIM) that allows K-bZIP to enhance its own SUMOylation and that of other cellular proteins known to interact with it, including the tumor suppressor proteins p53 and pRB [153]. In consequence, it has been postulated that K-bZIP acts as a viral encoded SUMO ligase that helps ensure the maintenance of the proper cellular environment needed for viral multiplication by triggering the SUMOylation and subsequent activation of p53, which in turn triggers cell cycle arrest in G1 [153].

iv) VP35: The VP35 protein encoded by Ebola Zaire virus (EBOV) is one of two EBOV viral proteins known to be involved in suppressing the type I interferon (IFN) response in the cell. The mechanism responsible for IFN inhibition was postulated to involve VP35's ability to bind to dsRNA therefore preventing retinoic acid induced gene I (RIG-I) activation [154]. However, a mutant form of VP35 incapable of binding dsRNA was found to retain its IFN blocking activity, suggesting the existence of an alternative mechanism for IFN inhibition by VP35. Type I IFN production is ultimately triggered by the transactivational activity of NF-κB and two additional transcription factors: Interferon regulatory factors 3 and 7 (IRF3 and IRF7, respectively). VP35 was demonstrated to interact with the SUMO ligase PIAS1, the E2 SUMO conjugating enzyme Ubc9, and IRF7. Furthermore, VP35's ability to interact simultaneously with all of these factors was shown to enhance the SUMOylation of IRF7 and IRF3. In turn, the enhanced SUMOylation of IRF7 and IRF3 was demonstrated to diminish their ability to transactivate type I IFN production, therefore leading to a substantial decrease in type I IFN production during EBOV infection [155]. In consequence, VP35 represents a viral protein that enhances the activity of a SUMO ligase as a way to neutralize the transcriptional activity of specific cellular factors, therefore leading to decreased type I IFN production and diminished cellular antiviral responses during infection, an outcome that favors viral multiplication.

Altogether, the four proteins presented above, encoded by four different pathogens, exemplify some of the most important interactions established between infectious organisms and the cellular SUMOylation system and provide a framework to understand the potential roles played by SUMO during influenza virus infection.

4.4. The beginning of the wrestling match: Initial insights into the relevance of the cellular SUMOylation system for influenza virus infections

Our laboratory was arguably the first in studying the potential interplay between the cellular SUMOylation system and influenza virus. Our initial studies on this topic, dating back to 2005, were motivated by the well established relevance of SUMO for the biological activities of numerous proteins encoded by DNA viruses [156]. The unifying theme at the time was that SUMO appeared to regulate numerous viral proteins targeted to the nucleus of the cell. Because influenza replication occurs in the nucleus of the infected cell, it seemed plausible that some influenza viral proteins would turn out to be SUMO targets. Our initial test of this hypothesis involved *in vitro* SUMOylation reactions in which ^{35}S-methionine labeled viral proteins produced in a coupled transcription/translation system were incubated with a fully purified reconstituted SUMOylation system. The data produced by these experiments were surprising and unexpected as they showed that most of the 9 viral proteins tested were SUMOylatable *in vitro*. The only viral proteins that were not tested were PB1-F2 and M2, and the only two proteins that did not appear to be SUMOylated were the two membrane viral proteins tested, HA and NA [157].

Although our personal experience has indicated direct correlation between *in vitro* SUMOylation and *in vivo* SUMOylation, it was necessary to demonstrate that the viral proteins identified as SUMO targets *in vitro* could also become SUMOylated when expressed in mammalian cells. This proved more challenging than expected, partially due to the limited pool of free SUMO normally present in the cell, and required the development of a set of dicistronic expression constructs capable of simultaneously inducing large increases in the cellular concentrations of SUMO accompanied by slight increases in the cellular pool of its conjugating enzyme Ubc9. The development and implementation of such dicistronic expression constructs allowed us to demonstrate that the non-structural influenza protein NS1 is a *bona-fide* SUMO target *in vivo*, being SUMOylated both, when over-expressed by transfection, as well as when expressed at normal physiological levels during viral infection. On the day this finding was published online, 14 November 2009, it constituted the first published report supporting the potential relevance of SUMOylation for influenza virus [158], and the dicistronic constructs described therein have subsequently been proven invaluable as key tools in numerous studies related to the SUMOylation of other cellular and viral proteins [157, 159-160].

Just one month after the publication of our report, further evidence supporting an important role for the cellular SUMOylation system during influenza virus infection was provided by two papers reporting the outcome of large scale screenings aimed at identifying cellular proteins required for efficient influenza virus infection. In the first report, published online on 21 December 2009, König et al. reported the identification of SUMO2, SUMO1, and SAE1 among the cellular genes whose down-regulation by RNAi in a human lung epithelial cell line (A549) led to a substantial decrease in viral transcription/translation, as assessed using a Renilla luciferase reporter system placed in substitution for the HA protein in a recombinant A/WSN/1933 H1N1 viral strain [92]. In the second report, published online on 24 December 2009, Shapira et al. identified Ube2I (i.e. Ubc9, the SUMO conjugating enzyme) as one of the cellular proteins capable of establishing direct physical interactions with the viral proteins PB1 and NS1 derived from the A/Puerto Rico/8/1934 H1N1 viral strain, and the NS1 protein derived from the A/Udorn/307/1972 H3N2 viral strain. In that report, the significance of those interactions, initially detected during the implementation of a large yeast two hybrid screening for cellular proteins capable of interacting with viral proteins, was further validated by using an RNAi approach [94]. Altogether, the two large scale screenings for cellular proteins required for efficient influenza virus infection confirmed the relevance of the SUMOylation system for influenza suggested by our initial studies.

4.5. Wrestling with the interferon response of the host: Relevance of the cellular SUMOylation system for the biological functions of the non-structural viral protein NS1

Almost exactly one year after the initial publication of our report on the SUMOylation of NS1, a collaborative effort involving personnel distributed across ten institutions in two different countries, China and Germany, led to the publication of a report, authored by Xu et al., on the SUMOylation of the NS1 protein of the highly pathogenic avian influenza A/Duck/Hubei/L-1/2004 H5N1 viral strain (published online on 3 November 2010) [161]. According to that report, the authors initially identified Ubc9 as a host-cell protein capable of interacting with a truncated form of NS1 (ending at position 162) in a yeast two hybrid screening executed with the goal of identifying novel host cell protein interactors for NS1. The authors then demonstrated that the H5N1 NS1 is SUMOylated *in vivo* when over-expressed by transfection, as were the NS1 proteins encoded by most viral strains tested, with the sole exception of the NS1 derived from the A/Sichuan/1/2009 H1N1 2009 pandemic strain. The authors also demonstrated that over-expression of the SUMO-deconjugating enzyme SENP1 abolished NS1 SUMOylation, and provided data indicative of NS1 SUMOylation during infection. Subsequent analyses mapped the SUMOylation site in the H5N1 NS1 at residue K221, but indicated that residue K219 could provide an alternative SUMOylation site when K221 was mutated [161].

One of the most important functions associated to NS1 during infection is its ability to neutralize the cellular type-I interferon (IFN) response. In the report by Xu et al., the authors compared the type I IFN-inhibiting activity of the wild-type (wt) NS1 with that of the non-SUMOylatable mutant and found a slight decrease in the non-SUMOylatable mutant's ability to neutralize the IFN response. Subsequent cycloheximide analyses indicated that the non-SUMOylatable NS1 appeared to have a substantial reduction in its stability, therefore accumulating to significantly lower levels in the cell. This property was then considered to be responsible for the non-SUMOylatable mutant's decreased ability to neutralize the type I IFN response. Finally, to study the potential effects of SUMOylation on viral growth, the authors developed a recombinant virus carrying a non-SUMOylatable NS1 in which K219 and K221 were changed to glutamic acid to prevent introducing mutations in NS2, which is encoded by a spliced transcript of the NS gene segment. The resulting mutant virus grew to almost identical titers as the wt virus, but exhibited a 10 fold decrease in viral production at 8 hours post-infection [161].

Recent data obtained by our group further supported the relevance of SUMOylation for NS1, although slight differences with the data presented in the paper by Xu et al. were observed. Such differences provide alternative mechanistic scenarios to explain the molecular effects of SUMOylation on NS1 function. First, our mapping analyses yielded somewhat different data: According to our findings (Santos et al., manuscript in revision), the primary SUMOylation site in NS1 is not residue K221 but residue K219, which shows partial conservation among different viral strains. Our analyses have also mapped a secondary SUMOylation site in NS1, located in residue K70, a residue that is almost perfectly conserved among all influenza A viral strains. Thus, to abrogate NS1 SUMOylation, it is necessary to simultaneously mutate both, K219 and K70. To this end we developed a double mutant form of NS1, hereafter referred to as NS1K70AK219A, in which both lysines were substituted by alanine. Second, protein stability analyses using cycloheximide also produced slightly different data: Despite numerous repeats, our experiments did not show differences between the stability of the non-SUMOylatable NS1K70AK219A mutant and that of wt NS1 (Santos et al., manuscript in revision). Therefore, our data indicates that SUMOylation does not appear to regulate NS1's stability. Finally, viral replication assays demonstrated that NS1's ability to become SUMOylated exerts more dramatic effects on viral multiplication (as evidenced by the viral titers produced during infection) than those observed by Xu. et al. During the execution of these experiments, we decided to prevent introducing mutations affecting NS2 in the virus carrying the NS1K70AK219A mutant form of NS1 by mutating the splicing acceptor site located in NS1 and moving it, together with a full copy of the second exon for NS2, downstream from the stop codon for NS1. This strategy had been previously developed and successfully implemented by Varble et al. and offers the advantage of allowing the independent manipulation of NS1 and NS2 while still allowing NS2 to be produced as a splicing product of the primary transcript transcribed off the NS gene segment [162]. The NS gene segment generated in this way, hereafter referred to as NS1K70AK219A~NS2wt, produces a non-SUMOylatable NS1 and a wt NS2. To allow proper comparison of growth characteristics in the absence of other potential effects due to the alterations introduced in the NS gene segment, we also developed an equivalent NS gene segment coding for wt (SUMOylatable) NS1, hereafter referred to as NS1wt~NS2wt. The resulting recombinant viruses generated with those NS gene segments, produced by reverse genetics, exhibited striking differences in growth: The virus carrying the NS1wt~NS2wt gene segment produced viral titers that were more than two orders of magnitude (i.e. 100 fold) higher than the virus carrying the NS1K70AK219A~NS2wt gene segment, therefore supporting a very important biological role for the SUMOylation of NS1.

To better understand the effects mediated by SUMOylation on NS1, in addition to producing the non-SUMOylatable form of NS1, we also developed an artificial SUMO ligase (ASL) specific for NS1 (hereafter referred to as NS1-ASL). This innovative tool allows NS1 SUMOylation to be dramatically increased in the absence of any other noticeable change in the SUMOylation of any other protein within the cell (Pal et al., manuscript in preparation). Using this tool we have recently demonstrated that a ~4 fold increase in the fraction of SUMOylated NS1 produces a 25% decrease in NS1's ability to block type I IFN production, whereas blocking NS1 SUMOylation (by introducing the K70A and K219A mutations) produces a 60% decrease in NS1's ability to inhibit type I IFN production. This intriguing observation suggests that there is an intrinsic optimal balance in NS1's SUMOylation levels, and that whenever such balance is disrupted, whether by increasing or decreasing the proportion of SUMOylated NS1 present in the cell, NS1's IFN blocking activity is diminished. A likely explanation for this model relates to SUMO's ability to modulate the protein interactions established by its targets. NS1 is known to interact with numerous viral and cellular proteins, potentially forming a large number of different protein complexes, each associated to specific roles mediated by NS1. More than one of such complexes may affect NS1's abililty to neutralize type I IFN production. For instance, a homo-multimeric NS1 complex might be ideal for coating the viral RNA, therefore preventing RIG-I activation, whereas a complex of NS1 and CPSF might be needed to down-regulate the production of mature cellular mRNAs, including those coding for type I IFNs. Then, it is possible that the levels of SUMOylated NS1 dictate the types of complexes formed by NS1 and their proportion, so that altering the levels of SUMOylated NS1 will affect NS1's function by altering the proportion and nature of the different complexes formed by NS1. Native gels performed with cell extracts derived from cells expressing either NS1wt or NS1K70AK219A, with and without co-expression of the NS1-ASL, have provided experimental support by this hypothetical model by demonstrating SUMOylation-dependent changes in the protein complexes formed by NS1 (Pal et al., manuscript in preparation).

Altogether, our data indicates that the molecular effects mediated by SUMOylation on NS1 are likely to be complex and multifactorial, and that a molecular characterization of the complexes formed by SUMOylated and non-SUMOylated NS1 will be needed to truly understand how SUMOylation affects NS1 function. Furthermore, our data also indicates that it will be necessary to explore in detail the effects of SUMOylation upon NS1 proteins derived from numerous viral strains, as it is likely that the differences observed between the data reported by Xu et al. and our own analyses may reflect strain-specific effects mediated by SUMOylation on NS1 function. Such differences may in turn reflect differences in the distribution of SUMOylation sites in NS1.

4.6. A SUMO-dependent matrix: Relevance of the cellular SUMOylation system for the biological functions of the viral matrix protein M1

An important addition to the history of the interactions established between the SUMOylation system and influenza virus was published online on 20 April 2011 by We et al. [163]. In their manuscript, Wu et al. reported a critical role for SUMO in viral assembly, mediated by the SUMOylation of the M1 protein. The study was initiated by experiments aimed at evaluating whether knocking down the cellular expression of Ubc9 by an RNAi approach affected influenza virus multiplication in Huh7 cells (a hepatoma cell line). Interestingly, cells exhibiting an almost complete knock-down of Ubc9 (achieved by transducing the cells with a lentivirus carrying an shRNA against Ubc9 followed by puromycin selection of the transduced cells) exhibited a decrease of two orders of magnitude in viral production when compared with cells transduced with a lentivirus lacking an Ubc9-specific shRNA. Subsequent analyses demonstrated that the changes in viral production were not mirrored by similar changes in viral protein synthesis. More surprisingly, vRNA accumulation within the Ubc9 knocked-down cells appeared increased, therefore suggesting a defect in viral release and a potential role for SUMOylation during viral maturation and assembly. The authors then focused their attention on M1, an important player in viral assembly, and found it to be SUMOylated at position K242 [163].

To determine the role of M1 SUMOylation during viral infection, the authors developed a recombinant A/WSN/1933 H1N1 virus carrying a non-SUMOylatable form of M1 containing a lysine to glutamic acid substitution at position K242, hereafter referred to as M1K242E. The lysine to glutamic acid substitution was chosen to prevent introducing any mutations on M2, the other protein encoded by the M gene segment. The mutant virus produced final viral titers two orders of magnitude lower than those produced by the wt virus. Interestingly, the cellular distribution of the NP protein appeared to be substantially altered in cells infected with the mutant virus, displaying a mostly nuclear localization even late during infection, a time when most of the NP signal is usually localized in the cytoplasm and in close proximity to the plasma membrane. However, according to the authors, the cellular localization of M1 was not affected. This suggested that M1 SUMOylation could potentially affect the nuclear export of vRNPs by enhancing their interaction with M1. A subsequent series of immunoprecipitation analyses showed that, in the presence of the non-SUMOylatable form of M1, the interactions between M1 and two proteins normally associated with vRNPs, PB2 and NP, were substantially decreased. This provided empirical support to the role of M1 SUMOylation in enhancing the interaction between M1 and vRNPs. Further support was provided by transmission electron microscopy data showing that, in cells infected with the mutant virus, a high number of empty virus-like particles and viral particles with abnormal morphology were produced, defects normally associated with a weak M1-vRNP interaction [163].

Altogether, the report by Wu et al. presented a very compelling story demonstrating a role for M1 SUMOylation in enhancing the interaction between M1 and the vRNP. We have also observed the SUMOylation of M1 in our own studies, a fact that we reported in our paper published online on 3 March 2011, although we did not succeed in mapping its SUMOylation site. It will be interesting in the future to determine the specific protein interactions that are modulated by M1 SUMOylation, as M1 is known to establish multiple interactions, not only with other viral proteins but also with cellular proteins. A molecular characterization of such interactions may help define new druggable targets in cellular proteins.

4.7. The future of the wrestling match: The potential relevance of the SUMOylation system for the development of innovative antiviral therapies

In addition to the unquestionable role played by SUMOylation for the NS1 and M1 viral proteins, described in the sections above, data generated in our laboratory supports the idea that the interactions between the cellular SUMOylation system and influenza virus are even more complex than already indicated. This statement is supported by two main findings: First, in addition to NS1 and M1, our analyses have demonstrated that other viral proteins, namely PB1, NP, NEP [157], PB2, and PB1-F2 (Santos et al., manuscript in preparation) are also SUMOylated during infection . Second, analyses performed looking at the global profile of cellular SUMOylation at different points post-infection have demonstrated that influenza infection causes a global increase in cellular SUMOylation, characterized by the appearance of two new SUMOylated proteins of ~70 kD and 52 kD [157].

Out of the new viral proteins identified as SUMO targets, our recent studies have already indicated that SUMOylation plays an important regulatory role for the viral polymerase subunit PB1, and ongoing analyses suggest that the same might be true for NEP (unpublished observations). This implies that, besides helping regulate NS1's IFN-neutralizing activity and M1's role in viral morphogenesis (two well established effects of SUMOylation on influenza infections as discussed above), the cellular SUMOylation system may also regulate PB1's role in viral transcription and replication, and NEP's role in the nuclear export of vRNPs. Our studies have demonstrated the existence of an optimal proportion of SUMOylated and non-SUMOylated NS1 that maximizes its IFN-inhibitory activity. It is likely that a similar optimal proportion between the SUMOylated and non-SUMOylated forms may also exist for all the other viral proteins targeted by the cellular SUMOylation system. This possibility emphasizes one important feature of the SUMOylation system that makes it an especially attractive target for the development of new antiviral therapies: Alterations affecting the activity of the SUMOylation system, whether increasing it or decreasing it, will affect the proportions of SUMOylated and non-SUMOylated forms of not just one but several viral proteins. This will likely result in pronounced alterations in the proportions of the various protein complexes made by each viral protein during infection, which will in turn decrease viral multiplication by affecting multiple stages of influenza's life cycle. Therefore, the SUMOylation system constitutes one cellular target whose disruption would likely have multiple damaging effects on viral multiplication without having immediate deadly consequences for the cell. Proof of principle for this idea has already been provided by two studies that have demonstrated substantial decreases in viral multiplication when the SUMO conjugating enzyme is targeted by an RNAi approach [92, 94]. From this perspective, it is conceivable that the ongoing NIH-sponsored efforts by other laboratories to develop drug-like specific inhibitors of the cellular SUMOylation system may, in the long run, yield a new generation of anti-influenza drugs, some of which may prove useful against other viral diseases as well.

Viruses have developed numerous strategies to gain control over the cellular environment of the host as a way to maximize their own fitness. Many of the cellular systems whose activity is increased during viral infections are purposely increased to facilitate viral multiplication. However, other cellular systems are increased as a way to neutralize viral infection, as exemplified by the large number of cellular genes that are turned on by the IFN response. Our analyses have demonstrated that influenza A infections produce a dramatic increase in the activity of the cellular SUMOylation system [157]. This has been demonstrated for a large number of viral strains and cell lines, and therefore is likely to represent a general feature of influenza A infections. We have also proven that the global increase in cellular SUMOylation requires the presence of a transcriptionally active virus, as UV inactivated viruses are unable to trigger it [157]. Additional analyses have also indicated that IFN stimulation is neither sufficient nor required to trigger the increase, as direct addition of recombinant IFN-β to uninfected cells does not result in a global increase in cellular SUMOylation, and cells lacking the ability to produce IFN (such as Vero cells) also exhibit the increase upon viral infection [157]. Although these findings strongly suggest that the global increase in cellular SUMOylation is triggered by a virus-dependent mechanism, it is uncertain whether the increase itself corresponds to a viral strategy to enhance viral growth, or a cellular attempt at neutralizing viral infection. It appears tempting to choose the first scenario, particularly because of the already demonstrated relevance of SUMOylation for a number of viral proteins [161, 163] and the demonstrated decrease in viral multiplication observed upon targeting Ubc9 by RNAi [92, 94]. However, at this point we consider that it is still possible that some of the SUMOylation events that are induced during infection may have antiviral effects. Our ongoing studies have already identified the minimal set of viral components required to trigger the global increase in cellular SUMOylation described above (Chacon, Santos, et al., manuscript in preparation), and recent data have revealed an unanticipated twist in the story. We are confident that further characterization of the molecular mechanisms involved in the global increase in cellular SUMOylation by influenza virus will lead to a new paradigm for the interactions established between viruses and the SUMO system.

5. Conclusions

IAV remains one of the most damaging viruses for humans. Our knowledge of the molecular mechanisms involved in viral transcription and replication has increased dramatically, and with it, we have also gained new insights into how the host cell is affected by the virus to enhance viral functions, and how cellular functions affect viral replication. However, numerous questions remain, particularly in areas related to the dynamic interplay that takes place between the numerous cellular systems affected by the virus and the viral proteins that trigger those effects. A better understanding of the interplay established between the virus and its host cell is likely to result in the development of new therapeutic agents for the treatment and prevention of complicated influenza infections, which is, in our opinion, one of the most urgent medical needs of our time due to the impending threat of new pandemics. Research started by our group about 7 years ago has began to unveil some of the multiple roles that the cellular SUMOylation system plays during the life cycle of IAV. The variety and significance of those roles for viral fitness identifies the SUMO system as one of the most promising targets for the development of novel broad-spectrum, host-cell targeted, anti-influenza therapies, which could also be applicable to the treatment of other acute viral diseases.

Author details

Andrés Santos** and Jason Chacón **
Department of Biological Sciences, The University of Texas at El Paso (UTEP), USA

Germán Rosas-Acosta*
Border Biomedical Research Center (BBRC), The University of Texas at El Paso (UTEP), USA
Department of Biological Sciences, The University of Texas at El Paso (UTEP), USA

* Corresponding Author
** These authors contributed equally to this work

Acknowledgement

We apologize for having to omit citing numerous invaluable research papers that have contributed enormously toward our understanding of influenza biology due to space and time limitations. We would like to acknowledge all past and present members of the Rosas-Acosta laboratory for their contributions to our research. The Rosas-Acosta's laboratory has been supported by start-up funds provided by the University of Texas at El Paso (UTEP), grant #0765137Y from the American Heart Association (South-Central Filiate), grant #1SC2AI081377-01 from the National Institutes of Allergy and Infectious Diseases (NIAID) and the National Institute of General Medical Sciences (NIGMS), National Institutes of Health (NIH), and grant #1SC1AI098976-01 from the NIAID, NIH, all to Dr. Rosas-Acosta. A.S. was supported by the RISE program at UTEP, which is funded by grant #R25GM069621-02 from the National Institute of General Sciences, Division of Minority Opportunities in Research (MORE), which administers research training programs aimed at increasing the number of minority biomedical and behavioral scientists. Research at the Rosas-Acosta's laboratory is also possible thanks to the support provided by The Border Biomedical Research Center (BBRC) and some of its associated facilities, specially the DNA Sequencing, the Biomolecule Characterization, and the Cell Culture Core Facilities. Support to BBRC is provided by grant #5G12RR008124 from the NIH.

6. References

[1] Palese, P. and M.L. Shaw (2007) Orthomyxoviridae: The viruses and their replication. In: Fields' Virology. D.M. Knipe and P.M. Howley, Editors. Lippincott Williams & Wilkins: Philadelphia. p. 1647-1689.

[2] Steinhauer, D.A. and J.J. Skehel (2002) Genetics of influenza viruses. Annu Rev Genet. 36: 305-32.

[3] Rossman, J.S. and R.A. Lamb (2011) Influenza virus assembly and budding. Virology. 411(2): 229-36.

[4] Noda, T., Y. Sugita, K. Aoyama, A. Hirase, E. Kawakami, A. Miyazawa, H. Sagara, and Y. Kawaoka (2012) Three-dimensional analysis of ribonucleoprotein complexes in influenza A virus. Nat Commun. 3: 639.

[5] Nayak, D.P., R.A. Balogun, H. Yamada, Z.H. Zhou, and S. Barman (2009) Influenza virus morphogenesis and budding. Virus Res. 143(2): 147-61.

[6] Shaw, M.L., K.L. Stone, C.M. Colangelo, E.E. Gulcicek, and P. Palese (2008) Cellular proteins in influenza virus particles. PLoS Pathog. 4(6): e1000085.

[7] Boulo, S., H. Akarsu, R.W. Ruigrok, and F. Baudin (2007) Nuclear traffic of influenza virus proteins and ribonucleoprotein complexes. Virus Res. 124(1-2): 12-21.

[8] Hale, B.G., R.E. Randall, J. Ortin, and D. Jackson (2008) The multifunctional NS1 protein of influenza A viruses. J Gen Virol. 89(Pt 10): 2359-76.

[9] Lin, D., J. Lan, and Z. Zhang (2007) Structure and function of the NS1 protein of influenza A virus. Acta Biochim Biophys Sin (Shanghai). 39(3): 155-62.

[10] Krug, R.M., W. Yuan, D.L. Noah, and A.G. Latham (2003) Intracellular warfare between human influenza viruses and human cells: the roles of the viral NS1 protein. Virology. 309(2): 181-9.

[11] Dudek, S.E., L. Wixler, C. Nordhoff, A. Nordmann, D. Anhlan, V. Wixler, and S. Ludwig (2011) The influenza virus PB1-F2 protein has interferon antagonistic activity. Biol Chem. 392(12): 1135-44.

[12] Varga, Z.T., I. Ramos, R. Hai, M. Schmolke, A. Garcia-Sastre, A. Fernandez-Sesma, and P. Palese (2011) The influenza virus protein PB1-F2 inhibits the induction of type I interferon at the level of the MAVS adaptor protein. PLoS Pathog. 7(6): e1002067.

[13] Neumann, G., M.T. Hughes, and Y. Kawaoka (2000) Influenza A virus NS2 protein mediates vRNP nuclear export through NES-independent interaction with hCRM1. EMBO J. 19(24): 6751-8.

[14] Veit, M. and B. Thaa (2011) Association of influenza virus proteins with membrane rafts. Adv Virol. 2011: 370606.

[15] Rossman, J.S., X. Jing, G.P. Leser, and R.A. Lamb (2010) Influenza virus M2 protein mediates ESCRT-independent membrane scission. Cell. 142(6): 902-13.

[16] Temte, J.L. and J.P. Prunuske (2010) Seasonal influenza in primary care settings: review for primary care physicians. WMJ. 109(4): 193-200.

[17] Thompson, W.W., D.K. Shay, E. Weintraub, L. Brammer, C.B. Bridges, N.J. Cox, and K. Fukuda (2004) Influenza-associated hospitalizations in the United States. Jama. 292(11): 1333-40.

[18] Thompson, W.W., D.K. Shay, E. Weintraub, L. Brammer, N. Cox, L.J. Anderson, and K. Fukuda (2003) Mortality associated with influenza and respiratory syncytial virus in the United States. Jama. 289(2): 179-86.

[19] Naghavi, M., P. Wyde, S. Litovsky, M. Madjid, A. Akhtar, S. Naguib, M.S. Siadaty, S. Sanati, and W. Casscells (2003) Influenza infection exerts prominent inflammatory and thrombotic effects on the atherosclerotic plaques of apolipoprotein E-deficient mice. Circulation. 107(5): 762-8.

[20] Horimoto, T. and Y. Kawaoka (2005) Influenza: lessons from past pandemics, warnings from current incidents. Nat Rev Microbiol. 3(8): 591-600.

[21] Oslund, K.L. and N. Baumgarth (2011) Influenza-induced innate immunity: regulators of viral replication, respiratory tract pathology & adaptive immunity. Future Virol. 6(8): 951-962.

[22] Enserink, M. and J. Cohen (2009) Virus of the year. The novel H1N1 influenza. Science. 326(5960): 1607.

[23] Hardy, C.T., S.A. Young, R.G. Webster, C.W. Naeve, and R.J. Owens (1995) Egg fluids and cells of the chorioallantoic membrane of embryonated chicken eggs can select different variants of influenza A (H3N2) viruses. Virology. 211(1): 302-6.

[24] Roose, K., W. Fiers, and X. Saelens (2009) Pandemic preparedness: toward a universal influenza vaccine. Drug News Perspect. 22(2): 80-92.

[25] Steel, J., A.C. Lowen, T.T. Wang, M. Yondola, Q. Gao, K. Haye, A. Garcia-Sastre, and P. Palese (2010) Influenza virus vaccine based on the conserved hemagglutinin stalk domain. MBio. 1(1).

[26] De Clercq, E. (2006) Antiviral agents active against influenza A viruses. Nat Rev Drug Discov. 5(12): 1015-25.

[27] (2006) High levels of adamantane resistance among influenza A (H3N2) viruses and interim guidelines for use of antiviral agents--United States, 2005-06 influenza season. MMWR Morb Mortal Wkly Rep. 55(2): 44-6.

[28] Fiore, A.E., A. Fry, D. Shay, L. Gubareva, J.S. Bresee, and T.M. Uyeki (2011) Antiviral agents for the treatment and chemoprophylaxis of influenza --- recommendations of the Advisory Committee on Immunization Practices (ACIP). MMWR Recomm Rep. 60(1): 1-24.

[29] Zurcher, T., P.J. Yates, J. Daly, A. Sahasrabudhe, M. Walters, L. Dash, M. Tisdale, and J.L. McKimm-Breschkin (2006) Mutations conferring zanamivir resistance in human influenza virus N2 neuraminidases compromise virus fitness and are not stably maintained in vitro. J Antimicrob Chemother. 58(4): 723-32.

[30] (2009) Update: influenza activity - United States, September 28, 2008--January 31, 2009. MMWR Morb Mortal Wkly Rep. 58(5): 115-9.

[31] (2009) Update: influenza activity--United States, September 28, 2008-April 4, 2009, and composition of the 2009-10 influenza vaccine. MMWR Morb Mortal Wkly Rep. 58(14): 369-74.

[32] Storms, A.D., L.V. Gubareva, S. Su, J.T. Wheeling, M. Okomo-Adhiambo, C.Y. Pan, E. Reisdorf, K. St George, R. Myers, J.T. Wotton, S. Robinson, B. Leader, M. Thompson, M. Shannon, A. Klimov, and A.M. Fry (2012) Oseltamivir-resistant pandemic (H1N1) 2009 virus infections, United States, 2010-11. Emerg Infect Dis. 18(2): 308-11.

[33] Ludwig, S. (2011) Disruption of virus-host cell interactions and cell signaling pathways as an anti-viral approach against influenza virus infections. Biol Chem. 392(10): 837-47.

[34] Shaw, M.L. (2011) The host interactome of influenza virus presents new potential targets for antiviral drugs. Rev Med Virol. 21(6): 358-69.

[35] Taubenberger, J.K., A.H. Reid, T.A. Janczewski, and T.G. Fanning (2001) Integrating historical, clinical and molecular genetic data in order to explain the origin and virulence of the 1918 Spanish influenza virus. Philos Trans R Soc Lond B Biol Sci. 356(1416): 1829-39.

[36] Tumpey, T.M., C.F. Basler, P.V. Aguilar, H. Zeng, A. Solorzano, D.E. Swayne, N.J. Cox, J.M. Katz, J.K. Taubenberger, P. Palese, and A. Garcia-Sastre (2005) Characterization of the reconstructed 1918 Spanish influenza pandemic virus. Science. 310(5745): 77-80.

[37] Taubenberger, J.K. and J.C. Kash (2011) Insights on influenza pathogenesis from the grave. Virus Res. 162(1-2): 2-7.

[38] Taubenberger, J.K., A.H. Reid, R.M. Lourens, R. Wang, G. Jin, and T.G. Fanning (2005) Characterization of the 1918 influenza virus polymerase genes. Nature. 437(7060): 889-93.

[39] Smith, G.J., J. Bahl, D. Vijaykrishna, J. Zhang, L.L. Poon, H. Chen, R.G. Webster, J.S. Peiris, and Y. Guan (2009) Dating the emergence of pandemic influenza viruses. Proc Natl Acad Sci U S A. 106(28): 11709-12.

[40] Claas, E.C., A.D. Osterhaus, R. van Beek, J.C. De Jong, G.F. Rimmelzwaan, D.A. Senne, S. Krauss, K.F. Shortridge, and R.G. Webster (1998) Human influenza A H5N1 virus related to a highly pathogenic avian influenza virus. Lancet. 351(9101): 472-7.

[41] Subbarao, K., A. Klimov, J. Katz, H. Regnery, W. Lim, H. Hall, M. Perdue, D. Swayne, C. Bender, J. Huang, M. Hemphill, T. Rowe, M. Shaw, X. Xu, K. Fukuda, and N. Cox (1998) Characterization of an avian influenza A (H5N1) virus isolated from a child with a fatal respiratory illness. Science. 279(5349): 393-6.

[42] Palese, P. and T.T. Wang (2012) H5N1 influenza viruses: facts, not fear. Proc Natl Acad Sci U S A. 109(7): 2211-3.

[43] Shortridge, K.F. (1992) Pandemic influenza: a zoonosis? Semin Respir Infect. 7(1): 11-25.

[44] Ungchusak, K., P. Auewarakul, S.F. Dowell, R. Kitphati, W. Auwanit, P. Puthavathana, M. Uiprasertkul, K. Boonnak, C. Pittayawonganon, N.J. Cox, S.R. Zaki, P. Thawatsupha, M. Chittaganpitch, R. Khontong, J.M. Simmerman, and S. Chunsutthiwat (2005) Probable person-to-person transmission of avian influenza A (H5N1). N Engl J Med. 352(4): 333-40.

[45] Herfst, S., E.J. Schrauwen, M. Linster, S. Chutinimitkul, E. de Wit, V.J. Munster, E.M. Sorrell, T.M. Bestebroer, D.F. Burke, D.J. Smith, G.F. Rimmelzwaan, A.D. Osterhaus, and R.A. Fouchier (2012) Airborne transmission of influenza A/H5N1 virus between ferrets. Science. 336(6088): 1534-41.

[46] Imai, M., T. Watanabe, M. Hatta, S.C. Das, M. Ozawa, K. Shinya, G. Zhong, A. Hanson, H. Katsura, S. Watanabe, C. Li, E. Kawakami, S. Yamada, M. Kiso, Y. Suzuki, E.A. Maher, G. Neumann, and Y. Kawaoka (2012) Experimental adaptation of an influenza H5 HA confers respiratory droplet transmission to a reassortant H5 HA/H1N1 virus in ferrets. Nature. 486(7403): 420-8.

[47] Osterholm, M.T. and N.S. Kelley (2012) Mammalian-Transmissible H5N1 Influenza: Facts and Perspective. MBio. 3(2).

[48] Octaviani, C.P., M. Ozawa, S. Yamada, H. Goto, and Y. Kawaoka (2010) High genetic compatibility between swine-origin H1N1 and highly pathogenic avian H5N1 influenza viruses. J Virol.

[49] Bukrinskaya, A.G., N.K. Vorkunova, G.V. Kornilayeva, R.A. Narmanbetova, and G.K. Vorkunova (1982) Influenza virus uncoating in infected cells and effect of rimantadine. J Gen Virol. 60(Pt 1): 49-59.

[50] Sugrue, R.J. and A.J. Hay (1991) Structural characteristics of the M2 protein of influenza A viruses: evidence that it forms a tetrameric channel. Virology. 180(2): 617-24.

[51] Maeda, T. and S. Ohnishi (1980) Activation of influenza virus by acidic media causes hemolysis and fusion of erythrocytes. FEBS Lett. 122(2): 283-7.

[52] Huang, Q., R.P. Sivaramakrishna, K. Ludwig, T. Korte, C. Bottcher, and A. Herrmann (2003) Early steps of the conformational change of influenza virus hemagglutinin to a

fusion active state: stability and energetics of the hemagglutinin. Biochim Biophys Acta. 1614(1): 3-13.

[53] Doms, R.W., A. Helenius, and J. White (1985) Membrane fusion activity of the influenza virus hemagglutinin. The low pH-induced conformational change. J Biol Chem. 260(5): 2973-81.

[54] Wu, W.W., Y.H. Sun, and N. Pante (2007) Nuclear import of influenza A viral ribonucleoprotein complexes is mediated by two nuclear localization sequences on viral nucleoprotein. Virol J. 4: 49.

[55] Wu, W.W. and N. Pante (2009) The directionality of the nuclear transport of the influenza A genome is driven by selective exposure of nuclear localization sequences on nucleoprotein. Virol J. 6: 68.

[56] Tarendeau, F., J. Boudet, D. Guilligay, P.J. Mas, C.M. Bougault, S. Boulo, F. Baudin, R.W. Ruigrok, N. Daigle, J. Ellenberg, S. Cusack, J.P. Simorre, and D.J. Hart (2007) Structure and nuclear import function of the C-terminal domain of influenza virus polymerase PB2 subunit. Nat Struct Mol Biol. 14(3): 229-33.

[57] Huet, S., S.V. Avilov, L. Ferbitz, N. Daigle, S. Cusack, and J. Ellenberg (2010) Nuclear import and assembly of influenza A virus RNA polymerase studied in live cells by fluorescence cross-correlation spectroscopy. J Virol. 84(3): 1254-64.

[58] Fodor, E. and M. Smith (2004) The PA subunit is required for efficient nuclear accumulation of the PB1 subunit of the influenza A virus RNA polymerase complex. J Virol. 78(17): 9144-53.

[59] Suzuki, T., A. Ainai, N. Nagata, T. Sata, H. Sawa, and H. Hasegawa (2011) A novel function of the N-terminal domain of PA in assembly of influenza A virus RNA polymerase. Biochem Biophys Res Commun. 414(4): 719-26.

[60] Ulmanen, I., B.A. Broni, and R.M. Krug (1981) Role of two of the influenza virus core P proteins in recognizing cap 1 structures (m7GpppNm) on RNAs and in initiating viral RNA transcription. Proc Natl Acad Sci U S A. 78(12): 7355-9.

[61] Biswas, S.K. and D.P. Nayak (1994) Mutational analysis of the conserved motifs of influenza A virus polymerase basic protein 1. J Virol. 68(3): 1819-26.

[62] Yuan, P., M. Bartlam, Z. Lou, S. Chen, J. Zhou, X. He, Z. Lv, R. Ge, X. Li, T. Deng, E. Fodor, Z. Rao, and Y. Liu (2009) Crystal structure of an avian influenza polymerase PA(N) reveals an endonuclease active site. Nature. 458(7240): 909-13.

[63] Dias, A., D. Bouvier, T. Crepin, A.A. McCarthy, D.J. Hart, F. Baudin, S. Cusack, and R.W. Ruigrok (2009) The cap-snatching endonuclease of influenza virus polymerase resides in the PA subunit. Nature. 458(7240): 914-8.

[64] Torreira, E., G. Schoehn, Y. Fernandez, N. Jorba, R.W. Ruigrok, S. Cusack, J. Ortin, and O. Llorca (2007) Three-dimensional model for the isolated recombinant influenza virus polymerase heterotrimer. Nucleic Acids Res. 35(11): 3774-83.

[65] Coloma, R., J.M. Valpuesta, R. Arranz, J.L. Carrascosa, J. Ortin, and J. Martin-Benito (2009) The structure of a biologically active influenza virus ribonucleoprotein complex. PLoS Pathog. 5(6): e1000491.

[66] Resa-Infante, P., M.A. Recuero-Checa, N. Zamarreno, O. Llorca, and J. Ortin (2010) Structural and functional characterization of an influenza virus RNA polymerase-genomic RNA complex. J Virol. 84(20): 10477-87.

[67] Area, E., J. Martin-Benito, P. Gastaminza, E. Torreira, J.M. Valpuesta, J.L. Carrascosa, and J. Ortin (2004) 3D structure of the influenza virus polymerase complex: localization of subunit domains. Proc Natl Acad Sci U S A. 101(1): 308-13.

[68] Shapiro, G.I., T. Gurney, Jr., and R.M. Krug (1987) Influenza virus gene expression: control mechanisms at early and late times of infection and nuclear-cytoplasmic transport of virus-specific RNAs. J Virol. 61(3): 764-73.

[69] Bouloy, M., S.J. Plotch, and R.M. Krug (1978) Globin mRNAs are primers for the transcription of influenza viral RNA in vitro. Proc Natl Acad Sci U S A. 75(10): 4886-90.

[70] Parvin, J.D., P. Palese, A. Honda, A. Ishihama, and M. Krystal (1989) Promoter analysis of influenza virus RNA polymerase. J Virol. 63(12): 5142-52.

[71] Cianci, C., L. Tiley, and M. Krystal (1995) Differential activation of the influenza virus polymerase via template RNA binding. J Virol. 69(7): 3995-9.

[72] Plotch, S.J., M. Bouloy, and R.M. Krug (1979) Transfer of 5'-terminal cap of globin mRNA to influenza viral complementary RNA during transcription in vitro. Proc Natl Acad Sci U S A. 76(4): 1618-22.

[73] Robertson, J.S., M. Schubert, and R.A. Lazzarini (1981) Polyadenylation sites for influenza virus mRNA. J Virol. 38(1): 157-63.

[74] Hsu, M.T., J.D. Parvin, S. Gupta, M. Krystal, and P. Palese (1987) Genomic RNAs of influenza viruses are held in a circular conformation in virions and in infected cells by a terminal panhandle. Proc Natl Acad Sci U S A. 84(22): 8140-4.

[75] Poon, L.L., D.C. Pritlove, J. Sharps, and G.G. Brownlee (1998) The RNA polymerase of influenza virus, bound to the 5' end of virion RNA, acts in cis to polyadenylate mRNA. J Virol. 72(10): 8214-9.

[76] Jorba, N., R. Coloma, and J. Ortin (2009) Genetic trans-complementation establishes a new model for influenza virus RNA transcription and replication. PLoS Pathog. 5(5): e1000462.

[77] Shapiro, G.I. and R.M. Krug (1988) Influenza virus RNA replication in vitro: synthesis of viral template RNAs and virion RNAs in the absence of an added primer. J Virol. 62(7): 2285-90.

[78] Robertson, J.S. (1979) 5' and 3' terminal nucleotide sequences of the RNA genome segments of influenza virus. Nucleic Acids Res. 6(12): 3745-57.

[79] Honda, A., K. Ueda, K. Nagata, and A. Ishihama (1988) RNA polymerase of influenza virus: role of NP in RNA chain elongation. J Biochem. 104(6): 1021-6.

[80] Vreede, F.T., T.E. Jung, and G.G. Brownlee (2004) Model suggesting that replication of influenza virus is regulated by stabilization of replicative intermediates. J Virol. 78(17): 9568-72.

[81] Cheong, H.K., C. Cheong, Y.S. Lee, B.L. Seong, and B.S. Choi (1999) Structure of influenza virus panhandle RNA studied by NMR spectroscopy and molecular modeling. Nucleic Acids Res. 27(5): 1392-7.

[82] Bae, S.H., H.K. Cheong, J.H. Lee, C. Cheong, M. Kainosho, and B.S. Choi (2001) Structural features of an influenza virus promoter and their implications for viral RNA synthesis. Proc Natl Acad Sci U S A. 98(19): 10602-7.

[83] Fodor, E., B.L. Seong, and G.G. Brownlee (1993) Photochemical cross-linking of influenza A polymerase to its virion RNA promoter defines a polymerase binding site at residues 9 to 12 of the promoter. J Gen Virol. 74 (Pt 7): 1327-33.

[84] Park, C.J., S.H. Bae, M.K. Lee, G. Varani, and B.S. Choi (2003) Solution structure of the influenza A virus cRNA promoter: implications for differential recognition of viral promoter structures by RNA-dependent RNA polymerase. Nucleic Acids Res. 31(11): 2824-32.

[85] Gonzalez, S. and J. Ortin (1999) Distinct regions of influenza virus PB1 polymerase subunit recognize vRNA and cRNA templates. EMBO J. 18(13): 3767-75.

[86] Robb, N.C., M. Smith, F.T. Vreede, and E. Fodor (2009) NS2/NEP protein regulates transcription and replication of the influenza virus RNA genome. J Gen Virol. 90(Pt 6): 1398-407.

[87] Perez, J.T., A. Varble, R. Sachidanandam, I. Zlatev, M. Manoharan, A. Garcia-Sastre, and B.R. tenOever (2010) Influenza A virus-generated small RNAs regulate the switch from transcription to replication. Proc Natl Acad Sci U S A. 107(25): 11525-30.

[88] Henderson, J.R. and F.J. Kemp (1959) Intracellular proteins associated with the synthesis of the influenza A virus. Virology. 9: 72-83.

[89] Mayer, D., K. Molawi, L. Martinez-Sobrido, A. Ghanem, S. Thomas, S. Baginsky, J. Grossmann, A. Garcia-Sastre, and M. Schwemmle (2007) Identification of cellular interaction partners of the influenza virus ribonucleoprotein complex and polymerase complex using proteomic-based approaches. J Proteome Res. 6(2): 672-82.

[90] Jorba, N., S. Juarez, E. Torreira, P. Gastaminza, N. Zamarreno, J.P. Albar, and J. Ortin (2008) Analysis of the interaction of influenza virus polymerase complex with human cell factors. Proteomics. 8(10): 2077-88.

[91] Hao, L., A. Sakurai, T. Watanabe, E. Sorensen, C.A. Nidom, M.A. Newton, P. Ahlquist, and Y. Kawaoka (2008) Drosophila RNAi screen identifies host genes important for influenza virus replication. Nature. 454(7206): 890-3.

[92] Konig, R., S. Stertz, Y. Zhou, A. Inoue, H.H. Hoffmann, S. Bhattacharyya, J.G. Alamares, D.M. Tscherne, M.B. Ortigoza, Y. Liang, Q. Gao, S.E. Andrews, S. Bandyopadhyay, P. De Jesus, B.P. Tu, L. Pache, C. Shih, A. Orth, G. Bonamy, L. Miraglia, T. Ideker, A. Garcia-Sastre, J.A. Young, P. Palese, M.L. Shaw, and S.K. Chanda (2010) Human host factors required for influenza virus replication. Nature. 463(7282): 813-7.

[93] Brass, A.L., I.C. Huang, Y. Benita, S.P. John, M.N. Krishnan, E.M. Feeley, B.J. Ryan, J.L. Weyer, L. van der Weyden, E. Fikrig, D.J. Adams, R.J. Xavier, M. Farzan, and S.J.

Elledge (2009) The IFITM proteins mediate cellular resistance to influenza A H1N1 virus, West Nile virus, and dengue virus. Cell. 139(7): 1243-54.

[94] Shapira, S.D., I. Gat-Viks, B.O. Shum, A. Dricot, M.M. de Grace, L. Wu, P.B. Gupta, T. Hao, S.J. Silver, D.E. Root, D.E. Hill, A. Regev, and N. Hacohen (2009) A physical and regulatory map of host-influenza interactions reveals pathways in H1N1 infection. Cell. 139(7): 1255-67.

[95] Karlas, A., N. Machuy, Y. Shin, K.P. Pleissner, A. Artarini, D. Heuer, D. Becker, H. Khalil, L.A. Ogilvie, S. Hess, A.P. Maurer, E. Muller, T. Wolff, T. Rudel, and T.F. Meyer (2010) Genome-wide RNAi screen identifies human host factors crucial for influenza virus replication. Nature. 463(7282): 818-22.

[96] Bortz, E., L. Westera, J. Maamary, J. Steel, R.A. Albrecht, B. Manicassamy, G. Chase, L. Martinez-Sobrido, M. Schwemmle, and A. Garcia-Sastre (2011) Host- and strain-specific regulation of influenza virus polymerase activity by interacting cellular proteins. MBio. 2(4).

[97] Tafforeau, L., T. Chantier, F. Pradezynski, J. Pellet, P.E. Mangeot, P.O. Vidalain, P. Andre, C. Rabourdin-Combe, and V. Lotteau (2011) Generation and comprehensive analysis of an influenza virus polymerase cellular interaction network. J Virol. 85(24): 13010-8.

[98] Huss, M., O. Vitavska, A. Albertmelcher, S. Bockelmann, C. Nardmann, K. Tabke, F. Tiburcy, and H. Wieczorek (2011) Vacuolar H(+)-ATPases: intra- and intermolecular interactions. Eur J Cell Biol. 90(9): 688-95.

[99] Guinea, R. and L. Carrasco (1994) Concanamycin A blocks influenza virus entry into cells under acidic conditions. FEBS Lett. 349(3): 327-30.

[100] Guinea, R. and L. Carrasco (1995) Requirement for vacuolar proton-ATPase activity during entry of influenza virus into cells. J Virol. 69(4): 2306-12.

[101] Muller, K.H., D.E. Kainov, K. El Bakkouri, X. Saelens, J.K. De Brabander, C. Kittel, E. Samm, and C.P. Muller (2011) The proton translocation domain of cellular vacuolar ATPase provides a target for the treatment of influenza A virus infections. Br J Pharmacol. 164(2): 344-57.

[102] Marjuki, H., A. Gornitzky, B.M. Marathe, N.A. Ilyushina, J.R. Aldridge, G. Desai, R.J. Webby, and R.G. Webster (2011) Influenza A virus-induced early activation of ERK and PI3K mediates V-ATPase-dependent intracellular pH change required for fusion. Cell Microbiol. 13(4): 587-601.

[103] Szul, T. and E. Sztul (2011) COPII and COPI traffic at the ER-Golgi interface. Physiology (Bethesda). 26(5): 348-64.

[104] Zhou, Z., Q. Xue, Y. Wan, Y. Yang, J. Wang, and T. Hung (2011) Lysosome-associated membrane glycoprotein 3 is involved in influenza A virus replication in human lung epithelial (A549) cells. Virol J. 8: 384.

[105] Marfori, M., A. Mynott, J.J. Ellis, A.M. Mehdi, N.F. Saunders, P.M. Curmi, J.K. Forwood, M. Boden, and B. Kobe (2011) Molecular basis for specificity of nuclear import and prediction of nuclear localization. Biochim Biophys Acta. 1813(9): 1562-77.

[106] Gabriel, G., A. Herwig, and H.D. Klenk (2008) Interaction of polymerase subunit PB2 and NP with importin alpha1 is a determinant of host range of influenza A virus. PLoS Pathog. 4(2): e11.

[107] Deng, T., O.G. Engelhardt, B. Thomas, A.V. Akoulitchev, G.G. Brownlee, and E. Fodor (2006) Role of ran binding protein 5 in nuclear import and assembly of the influenza virus RNA polymerase complex. J Virol. 80(24): 11911-9.

[108] Peterlin, B.M. and D.H. Price (2006) Controlling the elongation phase of transcription with P-TEFb. Mol Cell. 23(3): 297-305.

[109] Zhang, J., G. Li, and X. Ye (2010) Cyclin T1/CDK9 interacts with influenza A virus polymerase and facilitates its association with cellular RNA polymerase II. J Virol. 84(24): 12619-27.

[110] Braam, J., I. Ulmanen, and R.M. Krug (1983) Molecular model of a eucaryotic transcription complex: functions and movements of influenza P proteins during capped RNA-primed transcription. Cell. 34(2): 609-18.

[111] Luo, G.X., W. Luytjes, M. Enami, and P. Palese (1991) The polyadenylation signal of influenza virus RNA involves a stretch of uridines followed by the RNA duplex of the panhandle structure. J Virol. 65(6): 2861-7.

[112] Li, X. and P. Palese (1994) Characterization of the polyadenylation signal of influenza virus RNA. J Virol. 68(2): 1245-9.

[113] Landeras-Bueno, S., N. Jorba, M. Perez-Cidoncha, and J. Ortin (2011) The splicing factor proline-glutamine rich (SFPQ/PSF) is involved in influenza virus transcription. PLoS Pathog. 7(11): e1002397.

[114] Shen, H., X. Zheng, J. Shen, L. Zhang, R. Zhao, and M.R. Green (2008) Distinct activities of the DExD/H-box splicing factor hUAP56 facilitate stepwise assembly of the spliceosome. Genes Dev. 22(13): 1796-803.

[115] Luo, M.L., Z. Zhou, K. Magni, C. Christoforides, J. Rappsilber, M. Mann, and R. Reed (2001) Pre-mRNA splicing and mRNA export linked by direct interactions between UAP56 and Aly. Nature. 413(6856): 644-7.

[116] Schmidt, U., K.B. Im, C. Benzing, S. Janjetovic, K. Rippe, P. Lichter, and M. Wachsmuth (2009) Assembly and mobility of exon-exon junction complexes in living cells. RNA. 15(5): 862-76.

[117] Momose, F., C.F. Basler, R.E. O'Neill, A. Iwamatsu, P. Palese, and K. Nagata (2001) Cellular splicing factor RAF-2p48/NPI-5/BAT1/UAP56 interacts with the influenza virus nucleoprotein and enhances viral RNA synthesis. J Virol. 75(4): 1899-908.

[118] Bullock, A.N., S. Das, J.E. Debreczeni, P. Rellos, O. Fedorov, F.H. Niesen, K. Guo, E. Papagrigoriou, A.L. Amos, S. Cho, B.E. Turk, G. Ghosh, and S. Knapp (2009) Kinase domain insertions define distinct roles of CLK kinases in SR protein phosphorylation. Structure. 17(3): 352-62.

[119] Long, J.C. and J.F. Caceres (2009) The SR protein family of splicing factors: master regulators of gene expression. Biochem J. 417(1): 15-27.

[120] Shih, S.R., M.E. Nemeroff, and R.M. Krug (1995) The choice of alternative 5' splice sites in influenza virus M1 mRNA is regulated by the viral polymerase complex. Proc Natl Acad Sci U S A. 92(14): 6324-8.

[121] Shih, S.R. and R.M. Krug (1996) Novel exploitation of a nuclear function by influenza virus: the cellular SF2/ASF splicing factor controls the amount of the essential viral M2 ion channel protein in infected cells. EMBO J. 15(19): 5415-27.

[122] Alonso-Caplen, F.V. and R.M. Krug (1991) Regulation of the extent of splicing of influenza virus NS1 mRNA: role of the rates of splicing and of the nucleocytoplasmic transport of NS1 mRNA. Mol Cell Biol. 11(2): 1092-8.

[123] Robb, N.C., D. Jackson, F.T. Vreede, and E. Fodor (2010) Splicing of influenza A virus NS1 mRNA is independent of the viral NS1 protein. J Gen Virol. 91(Pt 9): 2331-40.

[124] Bier, K., A. York, and E. Fodor (2011) Cellular cap-binding proteins associate with influenza virus mRNAs. J Gen Virol. 92(Pt 7): 1627-34.

[125] Read, E.K. and P. Digard (2010) Individual influenza A virus mRNAs show differential dependence on cellular NXF1/TAP for their nuclear export. J Gen Virol. 91(Pt 5): 1290-301.

[126] Wisskirchen, C., T.H. Ludersdorfer, D.A. Muller, E. Moritz, and J. Pavlovic (2011) The cellular RNA helicase UAP56 is required for prevention of double-stranded RNA formation during influenza A virus infection. J Virol. 85(17): 8646-55.

[127] Fornerod, M., M. Ohno, M. Yoshida, and I.W. Mattaj (1997) CRM1 is an export receptor for leucine-rich nuclear export signals. Cell. 90(6): 1051-60.

[128] Akarsu, H., W.P. Burmeister, C. Petosa, I. Petit, C.W. Muller, R.W. Ruigrok, and F. Baudin (2003) Crystal structure of the M1 protein-binding domain of the influenza A virus nuclear export protein (NEP/NS2). EMBO J. 22(18): 4646-55.

[129] Chen, J., S. Huang, and Z. Chen (2010) Human cellular protein nucleoporin hNup98 interacts with influenza A virus NS2/nuclear export protein and overexpression of its GLFG repeat domain can inhibit virus propagation. J Gen Virol. 91(Pt 10): 2474-84.

[130] Ullrich, O., S. Reinsch, S. Urbe, M. Zerial, and R.G. Parton (1996) Rab11 regulates recycling through the pericentriolar recycling endosome. J Cell Biol. 135(4): 913-24.

[131] Eisfeld, A.J., E. Kawakami, T. Watanabe, G. Neumann, and Y. Kawaoka (2011) RAB11A is essential for transport of the influenza virus genome to the plasma membrane. J Virol. 85(13): 6117-26.

[132] Amorim, M.J., E.A. Bruce, E.K. Read, A. Foeglein, R. Mahen, A.D. Stuart, and P. Digard (2011) A Rab11- and microtubule-dependent mechanism for cytoplasmic transport of influenza A virus viral RNA. J Virol. 85(9): 4143-56.

[133] Momose, F., T. Sekimoto, T. Ohkura, S. Jo, A. Kawaguchi, K. Nagata, and Y. Morikawa (2011) Apical transport of influenza A virus ribonucleoprotein requires Rab11-positive recycling endosome. PLoS One. 6(6): e21123.

[134] Geiss-Friedlander, R. and F. Melchior (2007) Concepts in sumoylation: a decade on. Nat Rev Mol Cell Biol. 8(12): 947-56.

[135] Dohmen, R.J. (2004) SUMO protein modification. Biochim Biophys Acta. 1695(1-3): 113-31.

[136] Rosas-Acosta, G., W.K. Russell, A. Deyrieux, D.H. Russell, and V.G. Wilson (2005) A universal strategy for proteomic studies of SUMO and other ubiquitin-like modifiers. Mol Cell Proteomics. 4(1): 56-72.

[137] Vertegaal, A.C., J.S. Andersen, S.C. Ogg, R.T. Hay, M. Mann, and A.I. Lamond (2006) Distinct and overlapping sets of SUMO-1 and SUMO-2 target proteins revealed by quantitative proteomics. Mol Cell Proteomics. 5(12): 2298-310.

[138] Ulrich, H.D. (2008) The fast-growing business of SUMO chains. Mol Cell. 32(3): 301-5.

[139] Wilson, V.G. and P.R. Heaton (2008) Ubiquitin proteolytic system: focus on SUMO. Expert Rev Proteomics. 5(1): 121-35.

[140] Hay, R.T. (2005) SUMO A History of Modification. Mol Cell. 18(1): 1-12.

[141] Ganesan, A.K., Y. Kho, S.C. Kim, Y. Chen, Y. Zhao, and M.A. White (2007) Broad spectrum identification of SUMO substrates in melanoma cells. Proteomics. 7(13): 2216-21.

[142] Vertegaal, A.C., S.C. Ogg, E. Jaffray, M.S. Rodriguez, R.T. Hay, J.S. Andersen, M. Mann, and A.I. Lamond (2004) A proteomic study of SUMO-2 target proteins. J Biol Chem. 279(32): 33791-33798.

[143] Hilgarth, R.S., L.A. Murphy, H.S. Skaggs, D.C. Wilkerson, H. Xing, and K.D. Sarge (2004) Regulation and function of SUMO modification. J Biol Chem. 279(52): 53899-902.

[144] Gill, G. (2003) Post-translational modification by the small ubiquitin-related modifier SUMO has big effects on transcription factor activity. Curr Opin Genet Dev. 13(2): 108-13.

[145] Wilkinson, K.A. and J.M. Henley (2010) Mechanisms, regulation and consequences of protein SUMOylation. Biochem J. 428(2): 133-45.

[146] Bekes, M. and M. Drag (2012) Trojan Horse Strategies Used by Pathogens to Influence the Small Ubiquitin-Like Modifier (SUMO) System of Host Eukaryotic Cells. J Innate Immun. 4(2): 159-67.

[147] Chiocca, S., V. Kurtev, R. Colombo, R. Boggio, M.T. Sciurpi, G. Brosch, C. Seiser, G.F. Draetta, and M. Cotten (2002) Histone deacetylase 1 inactivation by an adenovirus early gene product. Curr Biol. 12(7): 594-8.

[148] Colombo, R., R. Boggio, C. Seiser, G.F. Draetta, and S. Chiocca (2002) The adenovirus protein Gam1 interferes with sumoylation of histone deacetylase 1. EMBO Rep. 22: 22.

[149] Boggio, R., A. Passafaro, and S. Chiocca (2007) Targeting SUMO E1 to ubiquitin ligases: a viral strategy to counteract sumoylation. J Biol Chem. 282(21): 15376-82.

[150] Chiocca, S. (2007) Viral control of the SUMO pathway: Gam1, a model system. Biochem Soc Trans. 35(Pt 6): 1419-21.

[151] Ribet, D., M. Hamon, E. Gouin, M.A. Nahori, F. Impens, H. Neyret-Kahn, K. Gevaert, J. Vandekerckhove, A. Dejean, and P. Cossart (2010) Listeria monocytogenes impairs SUMOylation for efficient infection. Nature. 464(7292): 1192-5.

[152] Izumiya, Y., T.J. Ellison, E.T. Yeh, J.U. Jung, P.A. Luciw, and H.J. Kung (2005) Kaposi's sarcoma-associated herpesvirus K-bZIP represses gene transcription via SUMO modification. J Virol. 79(15): 9912-25.

[153] Chang, P.C., Y. Izumiya, C.Y. Wu, L.D. Fitzgerald, M. Campbell, T.J. Ellison, K.S. Lam, P.A. Luciw, and H.J. Kung (2010) Kaposi's sarcoma-associated herpesvirus (KSHV) encodes a SUMO E3 ligase that is SIM-dependent and SUMO-2/3-specific. J Biol Chem. 285(8): 5266-73.

[154] Cardenas, W.B., Y.M. Loo, M. Gale, Jr., A.L. Hartman, C.R. Kimberlin, L. Martinez-Sobrido, E.O. Saphire, and C.F. Basler (2006) Ebola virus VP35 protein binds double-stranded RNA and inhibits alpha/beta interferon production induced by RIG-I signaling. J Virol. 80(11): 5168-78.

[155] Chang, T.H., T. Kubota, M. Matsuoka, S. Jones, S.B. Bradfute, M. Bray, and K. Ozato (2009) Ebola Zaire virus blocks type I interferon production by exploiting the host SUMO modification machinery. PLoS Pathog. 5(6): e1000493.

[156] Rosas-Acosta, G. and V.G. Wilson (2004) Viruses and Sumoylation. In: Sumoylation: Molecular Biology and Biochemistry. V.G. Wilson, Editor. Horizon Bioscience: Norfolk, U.K. p. 331-377.

[157] Pal, S., A. Santos, J.M. Rosas, J. Ortiz-Guzman, and G. Rosas-Acosta (2011) Influenza A virus interacts extensively with the cellular SUMOylation system during infection. Virus Res. 158(1-2): 12-27.

[158] Pal, S., J.M. Rosas, and G. Rosas-Acosta (2009) Identification of the non-structural influenza A viral protein NS1A as a bona fide target of the Small Ubiquitin-like MOdifier by the use of dicistronic expression constructs. J Virol Methods. 163(2): 498-504.

[159] Bueno, M.T., J.A. Garcia-Rivera, J.R. Kugelman, E. Morales, G. Rosas-Acosta, and M. Llano (2010) SUMOylation of the lens epithelium-derived growth factor/p75 attenuates its transcriptional activity on the heat shock protein 27 promoter. J Mol Biol. 399(2): 221-39.

[160] Liu, J., D. Zhang, W. Luo, Y. Yu, J. Yu, J. Li, X. Zhang, B. Zhang, J. Chen, X.R. Wu, G. Rosas-Acosta, and C. Huang (2011) X-linked inhibitor of apoptosis protein (XIAP) mediates cancer cell motility via Rho GDP dissociation inhibitor (RhoGDI)-dependent regulation of the cytoskeleton. J Biol Chem. 286(18): 15630-40.

[161] Xu, K., C. Klenk, B. Liu, B. Keiner, J. Cheng, B.J. Zheng, L. Li, Q. Han, C. Wang, T. Li, Z. Chen, Y. Shu, J. Liu, H.D. Klenk, and B. Sun (2011) Modification of nonstructural protein 1 of influenza A virus by SUMO1. J Virol. 85(2): 1086-98.

[162] Varble, A., M.A. Chua, J.T. Perez, B. Manicassamy, A. Garcia-Sastre, and B.R. tenOever (2010) Engineered RNA viral synthesis of microRNAs. Proc Natl Acad Sci U S A. 107(25): 11519-24.

[163] Wu, C.Y., K.S. Jeng, and M.M. Lai (2011) The SUMOylation of matrix protein M1 modulates the assembly and morphogenesis of influenza A virus. J Virol. 85(13): 6618-28.

Chapter 2

West Nile Virus: Basic Principles, Replication Mechanism, Immune Response and Important Genetic Determinants of Virulence

George Valiakos, Labrini V. Athanasiou, Antonia Touloudi, Vassilis Papatsiros, Vassiliki Spyrou, Liljana Petrovska and Charalambos Billinis

Additional information is available at the end of the chapter

http://dx.doi.org/10.5772/55198

1. Introduction

West Nile virus (WNV) was first isolated in Uganda (West Nile district) in 1937 from the blood of a native Ugandan woman [1] and until the end of the 20th century was considered a cause of viral encephalitis limited only in Africa and Asia. It became a global public health concern after the virus introduction in North America and especially New York in 1999 [2]. Before that, Romania had recorded the first large outbreak of West Nile neuroinvasive disease (WNND) in Europe in 1996, with 393 confirmed cases [3]. Since then, major outbreaks of WNV fever and encephalitis took place in regions throughout the world including America, Europe and Middle East, causing human and animal deaths. In the last decade, lineage 2 strains, considered of low virulence, have been introduced in Central and South Eastern Europe and were incriminated as causative agents of major human and animal disease outbreaks. A great number of WNV infections in humans occurred in 2010 and 2011 in Greece, with 363 laboratory confirmed cases and 44 deaths [4]. WNV lineage 2 strains were first detected from pools of *Culex* mosquitoes (strain Nea Santa-Greece-2010) [5] and a Eurasian magpie (strain magpie-Greece/10) [6] at the epicenter of the outbreak.

The unexpected high virulence of lineage 2 strains creates major concerns regarding the pathogenic potential of evolving and mutating WNV strains. The basic properties of WNV function will be presented focusing especially on the replication cycle, the pathogenicity mechanism as well as some important genetic determinants of virulence that have been recognized so far and can pose serious public health risks when present at various WNV strains.

2. Classification

West Nile Virus (WNV) is a member of the Flaviviridae family of single-stranded RNA viruses with linear non-segmented genomes. More than 58 members belong to the Flaviviridae family, whose name comes from the word "flavi", Latin for "yellow", because one of the most famous flaviviruses is the Yellow Fever Virus. Flaviviridae family is further divided in 3 genera: flaviviruses, pestiviruses and hepaciviruses. Pestivirus genus consists of 4 viral species that cause important animal diseases: Bovine Viral Diarrhea Virus type 1 and 2, Border Disease Virus and Classical Swine Fever Virus. The only member of the Hepacivirus genus is Hepatitis C virus. The Flavivirus genus is the largest with at least 53 species divided into 12 serologically related groups. Of these, the Japanese Encephalitis Virus (JEV) group (8 species) is the one with the most human-associated disease viruses; Japanese Encephalitis Virus, St. Louis Encephalitis Virus, Murray Valley Encephalitis Virus and West Nile Virus are four members of the JEV group that have been associated with widespread human and animal disease outbreaks [7]. The International Committee of Taxonomy of Viruses can be consulted for the most accurate update regarding nomenclature and taxonomy of all viruses at the species level [8].

3. Structure and genome

The WNV genome is a positive single stranded RNA of approximately 11000 nucleotides surrounded by an icosahedral nucleocapsid which is contained in a lipid bi-layered envelope, of approximately 50 nm in diameter (Figure 1). The genome is transcribed as a single polyprotein that is cleaved by host and viral proteases into three structural (C, prM/M, and E) and seven nonstructural (NS1, NS2A, NS2B, NS3, NS4A, NS4B, and NS5) proteins [9] (Figure 2). Recent studies also reported that a larger NS1-like (NS1') viral protein, which is often detected during infection, is the possible result of ribosomal frameshifting [10].

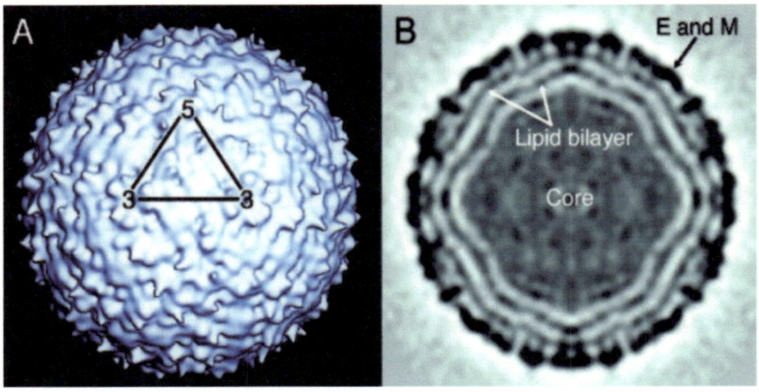

Figure 1. Structure of West Nile virus determined by cryo-EM. (A) A surface shaded view of the virion, one asymmetric unit of the icosahedron is indicated by the triangle. The 5-fold and 3-fold icosahedral symmetry axes are labeled. (B) A central cross section showing the concentric layers of density. Virion core, lipid bilayer and proteins E and M are indicated. Reprinted with permission from Science, 10 October 2003:248.DOI:10.1126/science.1089316.

The viral capsid is approximately 30 nm in diameter and consists of C protein dimers, the basic component of nucleocapsids, with the RNA binding domains located at the C- and N-termini separated by a hydrophobic region [11]. The hydrophobic regions of the C dimers form an apolar surface which binds to the inner side of the viral lipid membrane [12]. In immature virions, the lipid bi-layered envelope that coats the nucleocapsid contains 180 molecules each of E and prM proteins organized into 60 asymmetric trimeric spikes consisting of prM-E heterodimers [13]. The transition from immature to mature virions starts with the release of the N-terminal prepeptide from the prM protein after cleavage by a furin-like protease in the trans-Golgi compartment of the infected cell [14].

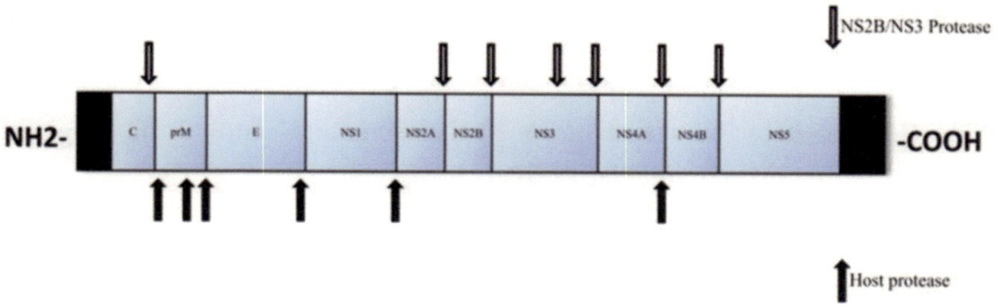

Figure 2. RNA genome of West Nile virus and site sites cleaved by host proteases and virus-encoded NS2B/NS3 protease.

Mature virions are characterized by the structural change, rotation and rearrangement of the 60 trimeric prM-E heterodimers to form 90 antiparallel homodimers with quasi-icosahedral symmetry that cover the lipid membrane [15, 16]. The E proteins are organized in 3 domains connected by flexible hinges [17]. Domain I (DI) is positioned at the central portion of the protein, linking together the other two domains. Domain II (DII) is a long domain containing a 13 residues long, glycine-rich, hydrophobic sequence that forms an internal fusion loop which is necessary for flaviviral fusion. Domain III (DIII) is an Ig-like fold that is thought to participate in interactions between virions and host factors associated with virus entry [18] (Figure 3).

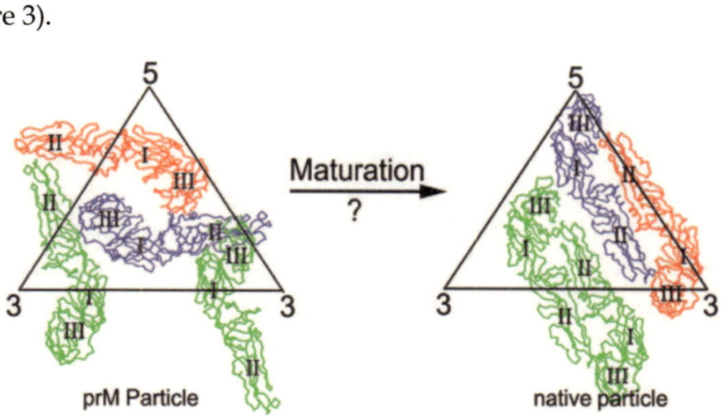

Figure 3. Diagram showing the structural rearrangement required for immature particles to become mature particles. The three independent E molecules per icosahedral asymmetric unit are colored green, red, and blue. The three domains in each E molecule are labeled I, II, and III. Reprinted with permission from EMBO J. 22(11):2604-13.

The viral nonstructural proteins are responsible for regulating viral mechanisms of transcription, translation and replication and attenuate host antiviral responses (Table 1). NS1 protein functions as a cofactor for viral RNA replication and is the only nonstructural protein that is secreted in high levels (up to 50 μg/ml) in the serum of WNV infected patients and has been connected with severe disease [19]. Many theories have been proposed regarding the contribution of NS1 to the pathogenic mechanism of WNV: it has been proposed to elicit hazardous autoantibodies [20], to contribute to the formation of various immune complexes circulating in the host organism [21], antibodies against NS1 to cause endothelial cell damage [22], or to minimize immune response targeting of WNV by decreasing recognition of infected cells by the complement system [23].

NS2A is a hydrophobic, multifunctional membrane-associated protein which plays an important role in RNA replication [24] and viral particles assembly [25, 26]. NS2A is also the major suppressor of beta interferon (IFN-β) transcription, thus inhibiting interferon response, one of the first lines of defense of the host [27].

NS2B is a cofactor required for NS3 proteolytic activity. NS3 is a multifunctional protein, with two distinct functional domains. The protease comprises the N-terminal amino acid residues of NS3, while the carboxylated terminus contains a helicase, a nucleoside triphosphatase and a RNA triphosphatase [28 - 31]. The NS3 trypsin-like serine protease is only active as a heterodimeric complex with its cofactor, NS2B. In the cytoplasm of infected host cells, this heterodimeric complex (NS2B-NS3pro) is responsible for post-translational cleavage of the viral polyprotein to release structural and non-structural viral proteins that are essential in viral replication mechanism and virions assembly. Cleavage takes place at the C-terminal side of two basic residues (e.g., RR, KK, and RK), a sequence motif that occurs at the junctions of NS2A/B, NS2B/3, NS3/4A, and NS4B/5. It also cleaves the viral polyprotein within the C-terminal region of protein C and protein NS4A as a necessary precursor to cleavage of prM and NS4B, respectively, by cell signalase in the lumen of the endoplasmic reticulum [28, 32]. The C-terminal of NS3 is characterized by the presence of motifs with homology to supergroup II RNA helicases, to a RNA-stimulated nucleoside triphosphatase (NTPase) and to a RNA triphosphatase (RTPase) [30, 33, 34]. The NTPase activity provides the chemical energy which is necessary to unwind RNA replication intermediates into forms that can be amplified by the NS5 RNA-dependent RNA polymerase [35, 36]. The RTPase dephosphorylates the 5′ end of viral RNA, before cap addition by the N-terminal methyl transferase region of NS5 [37]. RNA helicases travel along RNA in a 3′ to 5′ direction fueled by ATP hydrolysis; this movement opens secondary structures and displaces proteins bound to RNA [38]. Thus, together with the NS5 polymerase, with which NS3 is in tight association and interaction, the NS3hel plays an important role in flavivirus replication. However, a complete picture of the mechanism by which NS3hel associates with RNA template is not yet completely known.

NS4A, along with NS4B and NS2A, are the least known flavivirus proteins. The NS4A precise functional role has not been sufficiently characterized, although evidence suggests a role of "organizer" of the replication complex of flaviviruses. Its N-terminal is generated in the cytoplasm after cleavage by the NS2B-NS3 protease complex, whereas the C-terminal region (frequently designated 2K fragment) serves as a signal sequence for the translocation of the adjacent NS4B into the endoplasmic reticulum lumen. The 2K fragment is removed from the N terminus of NS4B by the host signalase, however a prior NS2B-NS3 protease complex activity at the NS4A/2K site is required [39]. Proteolytic removal of the 2K peptide also induces membrane alterations [40]. Recently NS4A was proven to act as a cofactor for NS3 helicase allowing the helicase to sustain the unwinding rate of the viral RNA under conditions of ATP deficiency [41]. NS4B colocalizes with viral replication complexes and proved to dissociate NS3 from single-stranded RNA, thereby enabling it to bind to a new dsRNA duplex, consequently enhancing the helicase activity and modulating viral replication [42, 43]. In addition, NS4A and NS4B, along with NS2A, as has already been referred, and NS5 proteins appear to inhibit the interferon-α/β response of the host [44-46].

Finally, NS5 is the C-terminal protein of the viral polyprotein and is the largest and most conserved of flaviviruses proteins. The N-terminal region of NS5 contains an S-adenosyl methionine methyltransferase (MTase) domain, part of the viral RNA capping machinery. The cap is a unique structure found at the 5′ end of viral and cellular eukaryotic mRNA, critical for both mRNA stability and binding to the ribosome during translation [47, 48]. The C-terminal region of NS5 contains a RNA-dependent RNA polymerase which is required for the synthesis of the viral RNA genome [49]. It was already mentioned that NS5 is in close interaction with NS3, constituting the major enzymatic components of the viral replication complex, which promotes efficient viral replication in close association with cellular host factors.

Non structural Protein	Function
NS1	Cofactor for viral RNA replication, pathogenic mechanism in early infection (decrease complement recognition)
NS2A	Viral RNA replication and virions assembly, Major suppressor of IFN-β transcription
NS2B	Cofactor for NS3pro activity, interferons antagonist
NS3	Serine protease, RNA helicase, RTPase, NTPase
NS4A	"Organizer" of replication complex, inhibitor of interferon α/β host response
NS4B	Inhibitor of interferon α/β host response, enhancer of NS3hel activity
NS5	Methyltransferase, RNA-dependent RNA polymerase, interferon antagonist

Table 1. Functions of West Nile virus nonstructural proteins.

4. Replication cycle

WNV has the ability to replicate in various types of cell cultures from a wide variety of species (mammal, avian, amphibian and insect) (Figure 4). The first step in the infectious cell entry involves the binding of E protein to a cellular molecule-receptor [50]. Several cell molecules have been proven to function as co-receptors for in-vitro virion attachment: WNV interacts with DC-SIGN and DC-SIGN-R in dendritic cells [51]. It has been documented to attach to the integrin αvb3, through DIII RGD/RGE sequence, which is an integrin recognition motif [52]. However a recent study showed that WNV entry does not require integrin αvb3 in certain cell types suggesting that receptor molecule usage is strain-specific and/or cell type-dependent [53].Rab 5 GTPase was found to be a requirement for WNV and Dengue Virus cellular entrance [54]. Laminin binding protein is also a putative receptor for the WNV, with proved high specificity and efficiency between LBP and DII of E protein [55, 56]. Many other attachment factors have been identified for flaviviruses, including CD14 [57], GRP78/BiP [58], 37-kDa/67-kDa laminin binding protein [58], heat-shock proteins 90 and 70 [59], and even negatively charged lycoaminoglycans, such as heparan sulfate, which are expressed in various cell types, though, for the latter, recent studies did not reveal specific binding of WNV with heparan sulfate [60].

After the viral attachment via the cellular receptors, WNV enters the cell through clathrin-mediated endocytosis [61]. It is characteristic that it was possible to inhibit WNV infection by treating cells with chemical inhibitors like chloropromazine [62] that prevent the formation of clathrin-coated pits, or by expressing negative mutants of Eps15 in cells. Eps15 is a protein involved in clathrin-coated pit formation [63]. The endosome environment is characterized by acidic PH, which triggers conformational changes of the E glycoprotein. The first step involves the disruption of the E protein rafts and dissociation of the E homodimers to monomers. An outward projection of DII takes place, and the fusion loop of DII is exposed to the target membrane. The E proteins insert their fusion loops into the outer leaflet of the cell membrane. Three E monomers interact with one another via their fusion loops to form an unstable trimer which is stabilized through additional interactions between the DI domains of the three E proteins [50, 64]. Next, DIII is believed to fold back against the trimer to form a hairpin-like configuration. The energy released by these conformational changes induces the formation of a hemifusion intermediate, in which the monolayers of the interacting membranes are merged. Finally, a fusion pore is formed and after enlargement of the pore, the nucleocapsid is released into the host cell. The viral RNA is released by the nucleocapsid with a yet unknown mechanism and is translated. The produced polyprotein is cleaved at multiple sites by the NS3 serine protease and the host signal peptidase within the lumen of the endoplasmic reticulum. At the same time, the viral RNA-dependent RNA polymerase copies complementary negative polarity (–) strands from the positive polarity genomic (+) RNA template, and these negative strands serve as templates for the synthesis of new positive viral RNAs. Studies showed that RNA replication can continue without protein synthesis, and that from a (+) strand RNA only one (-) strand RNA can be synthesized at a time, while from a (-) strand RNA multiple (+) strand RNAs can be simultaneously copied [65,66]. However virion assembly cannot take place if sufficient protein synthesis has not been performed: Each virion contains 180 copies each of E and prM structure proteins and only one genomic copy.

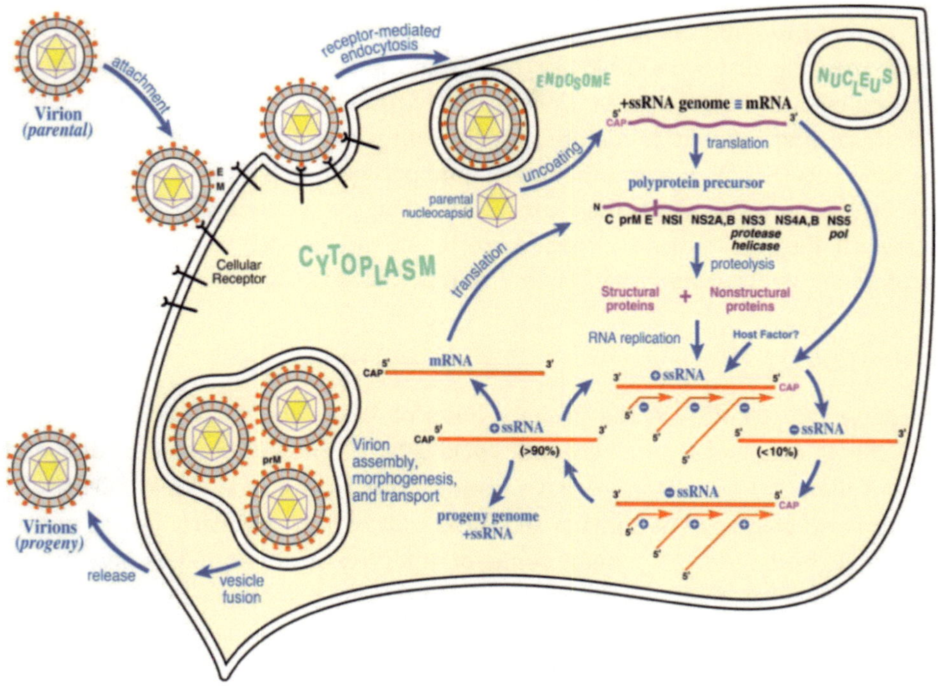

Figure 4. West Nile virus replication cycle. The virion is attached to the cellular membrane of thee host cell via the cellular receptors, and the envelope fuses with the membrane. The viral RNA is released by the nucleocapsid with a yet unknown mechanism and serves as mRNA for translation of all viral proteins and as template during RNA replication. Virion assembly and release of them to the extracellular milieu complete the replication cycle. Reprinted with permission from PNAS 2002, vol. 99 no. 18 11555-11557. Copyright 2002 National Academy of Sciences, U.S.A.

During West Nile virion assembly, C proteins bind to the newly replicated RNA and wrap around it to form an icosahedral shell. This nucleocapsid will be enveloped by cellular membrane derived from the endoplasmic reticulum and will bud into the lumen as immature virions on which E and prM proteins form 60 heterotrimeric spikes. Immature virions are then transported to the mildly acidic compartments of the trans-Golgi network triggering a rearrangement of E proteins on the immature virion; the lower pH induces a structural transition such that E proteins form 90 antiparallel homodimers on the surface of the virion [67] (Figure 4). Under acidic conditions, prM remains associated with the virion and protrudes from the surface of an otherwise smooth virus particle. This pH-dependent conformational change increases the susceptibility of prM for a furin-like serine protease [68].The pr peptide dissociates from the particle upon release of the virion to the extracellular milieu by exocytosis, which starts 10-12 h after cell infection. However, this furin processing of prM is rather inefficient and many virions still contain prM proteins even after their release to the extracellular milieu, which will reorganize back to prM/E heterodimers.

This inefficient and incomplete maturation leads to the secretion of a mixture of mature, immature and partially mature particles from flavivirus-infected cells. A high number of prM-containing particles have been described for WNV. Until recently, fully immature virions were considered to be unable to cause infection as they cannot undergo the structural rearrangements required for membrane fusion [69]. However, newer studies proved that even fully immature virions of flaviviruses can cause infection by antibodies [70, 71]. Regarding partially immature virions, multiple studies have shown that they can also be infectious [17, 72]. It seems that the mature part of these virions is responsible for cell binding and entry after which the further processing of remaining prM may take place inside the cell. Further studies are needed to estimate the "cut-off" regarding the number of prM proteins on viral surface that allow the viral particle to be infectious.

5. Epidemiology

Avian species are considered the primary hosts of West Nile virus, and in an endemic region, virus is maintained in an enzootic cycle between mosquitoes and birds [73]. Birds from more than 300 avian species have been reported dead from West Nile virus [74]. Disease can also be caused in humans and other mammals, particularly horses, considered as alternative hosts of WNV; main route of infection is through the bite of infected mosquitoes. However, the virus can also spread between individuals by blood transfusion and organ transplantation and few reports have also proposed the transmission from mother to newborn via the intrauterine route or via breast-feeding [75-77]. Most human infections remain asymptomatic, West Nile fever (a mild flu like fever) develops in approximately 20 to 30% of infected persons and West Nile neuroinvasive disease in <1% [78], characterized by encephalitis, meningitis, acute flaccid paralysis and even long-term neurological sequeale [79]. Nonetheless, horses and humans develop viremia levels of low magnitude (<10^5 PFU/ml) and short duration insufficient to infect mosquitoes and thus do not serve as amplifying hosts for WNV in nature [80]. On the contrary, various avian species, both migratory and sedentary, develop viremia levels sufficient to infect most feeding mosquitoes [81]. Hence, WNV is maintained in an enzootic cycle with wild and domestic birds being the main amplifying hosts and ornithophilic mosquitoes, especially of the Culex species, the main vectors. Moreover, local movements of resident birds and long-range travel of migratory birds may both contribute to the spread of WNV [82, 83]. Various studies have provided indirect evidence that WNV is transported by migratory birds, especially via their migration routes from breeding areas of Europe to wintering areas in Africa [84-87].

WNV strains are grouped into at least 7 genetic lineages [88] (Figure 5). Lineage 1 is the most widespread, containing isolates found in Europe, North America, Asia, Africa and Australia. This linage is further divided into at least two different clades: WNV-1a is found mainly in Africa, Europe, North America and Asia and is further divided in six evolution clusters [89].WNV 1-b contains the Australian Kunjin virus. A third clade containing Indian isolates is now classified as Lineage 5 [90]. Lineage 2 strains are mainly distributed in Sub-

Saharan Africa and Madagascar, but in the last decade they have been introduced in Europe. Lineage 3 contains a strain circulating in certain *Culex* and *Aedes* species mosquitoes in southern Moravia, Czech Republic, namely "Rabensburg virus", not known to be pathogenic to mammals [91]. Lineage 4 is represented by a strain isolated from *Dermacentor marginatus* ticks from the Caucasus [92]. A re-classification of Sarawak Kunjin virus as lineage 6 has been proposed as this strain is different to other Kunjin viruses. The African Koutango virus is closely related to WNV and a seventh lineage has been proposed for this strain. An eighth lineage has been proposed for WNV strains detected in *Culex pipiens* mosquitoes captured in Spain in 2006, which could not be assigned to previously described lineages of WNV [93].

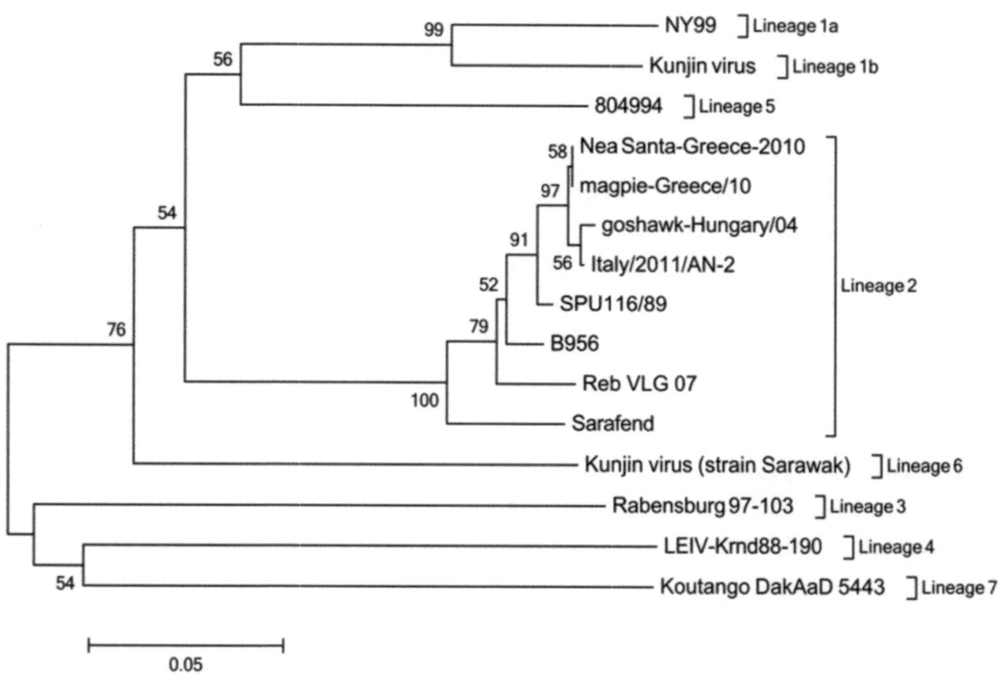

Figure 5. Phylogenetic tree of a 236-nt NS5 genomic region. Phylogenetic analysis based on a 236-nt NS5 genomic region of 15 West Nile virus strains, representatives of all recognized lineages, focusing on Lineage 2 strains circulating in South Eastern Europe. Analysis was performed using MEGA version 5. GenBank accession numbers and geographic origins of strains used in this analysis are: NY99 (AF202541, USA); Kunjin virus (D00246, Australia); 804994 (DQ256376, India); Nea Santa-Greece-2010 (HQ537483, Greece); magpie-Greece/10 (JQ954395, Greece); goshawk-Hungary/04 (DQ116961, Hungary); Italy/2011/AN-2 (JN858070, Italy);); SPU116/89 (EF429197, South Africa); B956 (AY532665, Uganda); Reb VLG 07 (FJ425721, Russia); Sarafend (AY688948, Israel); Kunjin virus/strain Sarawak (L49311, Malaysia); Rabensburg 97-103 (AY765264, Czech Republic); LEIV-Krnd88-190 (AY277251, Russia); Koutango DakAaD 5443 (L48980, Senegal). Neighbor-joining tree was constructed from a difference matrix employing the Kimura 2-parameter correction. One thousand bootstrap pseudo-replicates were used to test the branching (shown as percentages, with a cut-off value of 50%).

Lineage 2 was considered to be endemic in Sub-Saharan Africa and Madagascar, however, since 2004 strains have been observed in Hungary from birds of prey [94] and in 2007 in Russia from mosquito pools during a disease outbreak with 67 human cases [95]. In 2010 it caused outbreaks in Romania [96] and Greece [4] and in 2011 it was detected for the first time in Italy [97, 98]. The Greek and Italian strains showed the highest homology to Hungarian and South African strains, differing from the Russian lineage 2 strains detected in 2007. However, in Italy no major human disease outbreak occurred; only one human case was reported with mild clinical expression [97]. Genetic analysis of the Italian strains revealed the presence of histidine at 249 aa position of NS3, just like the Hungarian strains, in contrast to the Greek strains that contained proline at that position, the presence of which has been already implicated with high pathogenicity of lineage 1 strains [99].

6. Pathogenesis

Most of our knowledge regarding WNV dissemination and pathogenesis derives from the study in rodent models. After an infected mosquito bite, WNV infects keratinocytes and Langerhans cells [100,101] which migrate to lymph nodes resulting in a primary viremia [102]. Then the virus spreads to peripheral visceral organs like kidney and spleen where a new replication stage occurs, in epithelium cells and macrophages respectively [103]. Depending on the level of viremia, the peak of which comes at day 3 p.i. in mice, the virus may cross the blood-brain barrier (BBB) and enter the central nervous system (CNS), causing meningo-encephalitis. Various ways have been proposed for WNV entry to CNS; TNF-a mediated change in endothelial cell permeability have been proposed to facilitate CNS entry [104], as well as infection of olfactory neurons and spread to the olfactory bulb [105]. Other ways involve direct axonal retrograde transport from infected peripheral neurons [106] or transport of the virus by infected immune cells trafficking to the CNS [107]. WNV infects neurons in various parts of the CNS causing loss of architecture, degeneration and cell death. In a later stage mononuclear cells infiltrate the infected regions although it is not really clear if they help stop infection or contribute to pathogenesis destroying infected cells and releasing cytokines [108]. Infection and injury of brain stem, hippocampal and spinal cord is observed in both humans and rodents that succumb to the disease. Persistence of WNV in mice was found to be tissue dependent. Infectious virus could persist as long as 4 months p.i., especially in mice that did not exhibit disease during acute infection and especially in the skin and spinal cord [109]. This persistence may also occur in humans after mild febrile illness or subclinical infections; 3% of WNV-positive blood donors were found to have detectable WNV RNA in blood between 40 and 104 days after their index donation [110].

In wild birds, less is known regarding pathogenesis of WNV. The virus has been detected by histology and RT-PCR in various tissues e.g. brain, liver, lungs, heart, spleen and kidneys of various avian species e.g. crows, blue jays, goshawks, magpies [111, 112, 94, 6]. Various avian species were found to be viremic for 6 days post inoculation and viremic titers high enough to transmit the virus to mosquitoes via their bites [113]. In wild birds, infectious WNV was detected for as long as 6 weeks in tissues [114,115]. However it is important to clarify that immune response, virulence and viral persistence is to a great degree species dependent, with great variations among various avian species in different geographical areas, as well as strain dependent, implicating various genetic determinants of virulence.

7. Immune response

Immune response of animals and humans to WNV infection is divided to innate and adaptive.

Innate response includes interferons, complement and innate cellular immunity

Interferons type I (IFN-α and IFN-β), type II (IFN-γ), and type III (IFN- λ) IFNs play an essential protective role limiting infection of many viruses. IFN-α/β is produced by most of the cells following viral infection and induces an antiviral state to the cell, "activating" the relevant genes. It also creates a linkage between innate and adaptive immune responses by various mechanisms e.g. activation of B and T cells or dendritic-cell maturation [116, 117, 118]. IFN-γ is produced by $\gamma\delta$ T cells, $CD8^+$ T cells, and natural killer cells and limits early viral dissemination to the CNS through several mechanisms [119, 120]. WNV has evolved various countermeasures, at least 6 different mechanisms, against interferons function [121]. Hence, IFN administration cannot be considered of significant therapeutic importance for WNV disease control [122].

Several nucleic acid sensors e.g. TLR3, cytoplasmic dsRNA, RIG-I and MDA5 bind to viral RNA and activate transcription factors like IRF3 and IRF7 as well as IFN-stimulated genes [123-126].

Complement is a system of proteins in serum and molecules on cell surface that recognize pathogens and induce pathogen clearance. Three pathways exist for complement activation the classical, the lectin and alternative pathways, which are initiated by binding of C1q, mannan-binding lectins or hydrolysis of C3 respectively. All three pathways have been found to be important for controlling WNV lethal infections [127- 129].

There is data suggesting that macrophages and dendritic cells may directly inhibit WNV. Macrophages can control infection through cytokine and chemokine secretion, enhanced antigen presentation and direct viral clearance [130]. $\gamma\delta$ T cells also limit WNV infection in an early stage [131].

Adaptive response includes humoral and cellular response

Humoral immunity plays a vital role in protection from WNV infection. Experimental studies demonstrated complete lethality of B-cell-deficient and $IgM^{-/-}$ mice infected with WNV, whereas they were protected by transfer of immune sera [132,133]. IgM titers at day 4 p.i. could predict the disease outcome at prospective experiments. IgG can also protect from infection, however, in primary infection their role is less vital: Being produced after days 6-8, the disease outcome has been determined, since both viral shedding to CNS and clearance from tissues have already occurred [132, 134]. The vast majority of neutralizing antibodies are directed against all three domains of E protein. However the most potent neutralizing antibodies are directed on DIII possibly inhibiting viral fusion at post-attachment stage [135, 136]. In humans, antibodies against prM have also been recognized but with limited neutralizing activity [70, 137, 138]. Antibody neutralization is a procedure where multiple antibodies, above an estimated threshold "manage" to neutralize the virion's activity and render it non-infectious. This threshold was estimated to be 30 antibodies per virion for a highly accessible epitope of DIII of E protein [139-141]. It is important, however, to understand the following aspects: The level of neutralizing antibodies does not always correlate with protection against WNV. WNV have 180 E proteins on their surface. Steric phenomena because of the dense icosahedral arrangements of these proteins do not allow the equivalent display of all the epitopes. There are also many structurally distinct epitopes, not easily accessible to certain neutralizing antibodies. It is characteristic that studies showed a reduction of the neutralizing ability of antibodies correlated to the maturation state of WNV: Maturation reduces the accessibility of some of the epitopes on the virion [17]. Thus, these antibodies cannot efficiently neutralize the virus even if at high levels of concentration. This can lead to completely different result: Antibody dependent enhancement (ADE) of infection is possible in cells bearing activating Fc-γ receptors [141, 142] and thus a mild infection with sufficient levels of antibodies can become even life-threatening due to the inability of the antibodies to neutralize the virions.

Antibodies against NS1, a protein secreted in the serum of patients during acute phase of disease and expressed on the surface of infected cells considered to be a cofactor in virus replication, have been found to be non-neutralizing but protecting through both Fc-γ receptor-dependent and independent mechanisms [143].

T lymphocytes (part of cellular response mechanism) have been demonstrated to be vital for the protection against WNV infection. Recognizing an infected cell through the viral antigen fragments associated with MHC class I molecules on the infected cells' surface, cytotoxic ($CD8^+$) T cells secrete cytokines and lyse the cells directly (perforin, granzymes A and B) or indirectly via Fas-Fas ligand interactions [144, 145]. Studies showed that for the protection against lineage I, perforin played the most important role and, in contrast, lineage II strain Sarafend was controlled more efficiently by granzymes [146, 147]. $CD4^+$ T cells contribute through multiple mechanisms, and preliminary data suggest that $CD4^+$ T cells restrict pathogenesis in vivo [148]. Except IFN–α/β, T-cell immune response is extremely essential regarding the control of WNV in the CNS, their presence being correlated with virus clearance [146, 149, 150]. WNV infection induces the secretion of the chemokine CXCL10 from neurons, recruiting effector $CD8^+$ T cells via the chemokine receptor CXCR3 [151].Expression of chemokine receptor CCR5 and its ligand CCL5 is up-regulated by WNV and is associated with CNS infiltration of $CD4^+$ and $CD8^+$ T cells, $NK1.1^+$ and macrophages expressing the receptor [152].

All the above data provide solid evidence that a combination of various aspects of both innate and adaptive immune response cooperate to control WNV infection in the periphery and CNS.

8. Genetic determinants of virulence

Various studies especially in the last decade have recognized a variety of genetic determinants of virulence for West Nile virus strains. Specific mutations have been found to attenuate or strengthen virus pathogenicity via various mechanisms. Those that have been found to be the most important will be reported here, focusing on the ones that seem to have major impact on the replication mechanisms of WNV.

Mutations at the Envelope protein at residues 154 to 156, which abolished the N-linked glycosylation motif (N-Y-S/T) was proved to attenuate virus pathogenicity in mouse models [153]; these mutations seem to alter the protein such that it cannot be recognized by oligosaccharyl-transferase, thus glycan loss is caused [154]. This glycosylation motif has been recognized to various flaviviruses and spatially is located in close proximity to the center of the fusion peptide of DII of E protein, and thus is considered to increase the stability of the protein to a fusion-active form even at high temperatures [155, 156]. This proved to be really important for the multiplication of the virus to avian cell and animal models: results showed that E glycosylated WNV variants multiplied more efficiently to avian cell cultures and at high temperatures, causing at the same time high viremic titers and pathogenicity to chicks [157]. Most of the Lineage I virulent strains as well as recent virulent Lineage II strains associated with the Greek outbreak carry the N-glycosylation site, suggesting it a prerequisite for the efficient circulation and amplification of the virus in a mosquito-avian transmission cycle [158, Valiakos et al. unpublished data]. Of course it is possible that E glycosylation affects other aspects of the WNV replication cycle as well such as target cell tropism, virion assembly and release etc.

We have already referred to the NS4B protein proven dual role of involvement to virus replication mechanism (enhances helicase activity) and evasion of host innate immune defense (inhibits IFN α/β response). Studies proved that substitution of cysteine (an amicoacid which is often critical for the proper function of a protein) with serine at position 102 of NS4B, (Cys102Ser) leads to sensitivity to high temperatures as well as attenuation of the neuroinvasive and neurovirulent phenotypes in mice [159]. It was determined previously that the first 125 amino acids of the N-terminal of NS4B protein of flaviviruses are sufficient for the inhibition of IFN-α/β signaling [160]. Hence, this mutation which is located in this region of WNV may attenuate the viral ability to inhibit IFN signaling. Attenuation of the viral pathogenicity, characterized by lower viremia levels and no lethality to mice, was caused by a P38G mutation in the NS4B protein [161]; this was proven to be related to an induce of higher innate and adaptive immune response in mice, with higher type I IFNs and IL-1β levels and stronger memory and effector T cells responses. An adaptive mutation (E249G) in the NS4B gene resulted in reduced in-cell viral RNA synthesis, probably affecting the involvement of NS4B to the virus replication mechanism [162].

NS2A protein, as already stated, plays important role in RNA replication and viral particles assembly, and is also the major suppressor of IFN-β transcription. It was found that an A30P mutation of a Kunjin subtype WNV strain resulted in a reduced ability of the virus to inhibit IFN response, leading to increased levels of IFNs synthesis [27]. However this mutation implemented in North American Lineage 1 strains did not cause significant changes to phenotype indicating that in many cases the effect of mutations under study can be strain-specific. D73H and M108K were mutations found to be related to poor replication and non mortality to mice [163].

NS3 protein includes the serine protease at the N-terminal and the RNA helicase, an NTPase and an RTPase at the C-terminal. The introduction of a T249P in North American Linage 1 strain was found to be sufficient to generate a phenotype virulent to American crows [99]. A H249P mutation is considered to be the main cause of increased virulence of Lineage 2 strain that caused the major WNV disease outbreak in 2010-2011, in Greece. Only the Greek sequences, detected in mosquito pools, corvids and chickens [5, 164, Valiakos et al. unpublished data] contains proline at this locus, while all other Lineage 2 strains contain histidine. The exact mechanism through which this mutation increases the pathogenicity of WNV is unknown, believed though to be related to increased replication rate caused by an enhancement in RNA helicase function; hence, the virus may surpass bird viremia thresholds required for infection of many mosquito species vectors (> 10^5 PFU/ml. However, recent studies on European Lineage 1 strains Morocco/2003 and Spain/2007 proved that the first was more pathogenic in a mouse model than the second; Morocco/2003 contains a T and Spain/2007 a P at 249 aa position. Hence, a proline residue in position 249 of the NS3 position is not sufficient to enhance virulence, at least in certain cases [165, 166]. Another study detected a potential role of a S365G mutation to enhance viral replication, by lowering the requirement of ATP for ATPase activity, thus allowing the RNA helicase to sustain the unwinding rate of viral RNA under conditions of ATP deficiency [167].

The function of the hydrophobic 2K peptide that spans the ER membrane between NS4A and NS4B remains largely unknown. It is believed that it acts as signal sequence for the translocation of NS4B into the ER lumen. It is removed from the N-terminus of NS4B by a host ER signalase. 2K-V9M mutant virus generates higher viral titers in Oas1b-expressing cells than the wild type virus. The exact mechanism by which the 2K-V9M substitution enables WNV resistance to antiviral action of Oas1bis unknown [167].

Theoretically, substitutions of hydrophobic to hydrophilic amino acids and vice versa as well as substitutions of glycine, proline and cysteine residues are considered to have a potential effect on the secondary structure of proteins. A study performed on Lineage 2 strains of low and high virulence recognized this kind of substitutions at NS3 (S160A and R298G), NS4A (A79T) and NS5 protein (T614P, M625R, M626R) that were present at high virulent strains [168].

9. Conclusions

West Nile virus is considered a serious public health threat, especially for high risk groups (very young and elderly, imunocompromised). Currently there has not been established any antiviral treatment to WNV infections; only supportive care may be administered. Vaccine development is still at an early stage for humans. Hence, preventive measures rely still on reduction of mosquito populations and minimizing vector-host contact. Various diagnostic techniques have been developed the last decades, both molecular and serological, trying to minimize the difficulties arisen from other cross-reactive closely related flaviviruses. Data presented here prove the complexity of the host-virus interaction: Specific host-pathogen-vector interface, cellular tropism, viral structure diversity regarding maturation, immune system recognition and response, genetic diversity are all factors characterized by great variation rendering WNV control extremely difficult. Continuous studies are being demanded to understand the extent of this complexity to further elucidate biological relationships among host, vector and virus that will lead to improved disease control. As more is learned about the biological characteristics of WNV infection, one continuing objective will be to relate this knowledge to the clinical features of disease. An important viral-host determinant is virus attachment, mediated by cellular receptor and allowing subsequent infection. Host defensive behaviors that could affect virus acquisition and transmission should be also further studied. This may help in the design and implementation of more efficient and cost-effective control strategies since introduction of WN virus is an ongoing risk and reality. The ultimate challenge will be to apply the knowledge gained in understanding viral replication and unraveling the complexity leading to pathogenesis in order to prevent and control West Nile virus and its severe manifestations.

Author details

George Valiakos, Labrini V. Athanasiou, Antonia Touloudi, Vassilis Papatsiros, Vassiliki Spyrou, Liljana Petrovska and Charalambos Billinis
Faculty of Veterinary Medicine, School of Health Sciences, University of Thessaly, Greece

Acknowledgement

The research leading to these results received partial funding from the European Union Seventh Framework Programme (2007-2013) under grant agreement no. 222633 (WildTech).

10. References

[1] Smithburn KC, Hughes TP, Burke AW, Paul JH (1940) A Neurotropic Virus Isolated from the Blood of a Native of Uganda. Am. J. Trop. Med. Hyg. s1-20(4):471-92.
[2] Lanciotti RS, Roehrig JT, Deubel V, Smith J, Parker M, Steele K, et al. (1999) Origin of the West Nile Virus Responsible for an Outbreak of Encephalitis in the Northeastern United States. Science. 286(5448):2333-7.
[3] Tsai TF, Popovici F, Cernescu C, Campbell GL, Nedelcu NI (1998) West Nile Encephalitis Epidemic in Southeastern Romania. Lancet. 352(9130):767-71.
[4] Hellenic Centre for Disease Control and Prevention (HCDCP) [homepage on the Internet]. Greece, Ministry of Health and Social Solidarity [updated 2012 April 7; cited 2012 Apr 7]. Available from: http://www.keelpno.gr/en-us/home.aspx

[5] Papa A, Xanthopoulou K, Gewehr S, Mourelatos S (2011) Detection of West Nile virus lineage 2 in mosquitoes during a human outbreak in Greece. Clin. Microbiol. Infect. 17(8):1176-80.

[6] Valiakos G, Touloudi A, Iacovakis C, Athanasiou L, Birtsas P, Spyrou V, et al. (2011) Molecular detection and phylogenetic analysis of West Nile virus lineage 2 in sedentary wild birds (Eurasian magpie), Greece, 2010. Euro Surveill. 16(18): pii=19862.

[7] Schweitzer BK, Chapman NM, Iwen PC (2009) Overview of the Flaviviridae with an emphasis on the Japanese Encephalitis Group viruses. Lab Medicine 40(8):493-9.

[8] International Committee on Taxonomy of Viruses [homepage on the Internet]. USA, Virology Division of the International Union of Microbiological Societies [updated 2012 February 12; cited 2012 Apr 6] Available from: http://ictvonline.org/index.asp

[9] Chambers TJ, Hahn CS, Galler R, Rice CM (1990) Flavivirus genome organization, expression, and replication. Annu. Rev. Microbiol. 44:649-88.

[10] Melian EB, Hinzman E, Nagasaki T, Firth AE, Wills NM, Nouwens AS, et al. (2010) NS1′ of flaviviruses in the Japanese Encephalitis virus serogroup is a product of ribosomal frameshifting and plays a role in viral neuroinvasiveness. J. Virol. 84(3):1641-7.

[11] Diamond MS, Brinton MA (2009) Molecular biology of West Nile virus In: West Nile Encephalitis Virus Infection. Springer. pp. 97-136.

[12] Ma L, Jones CT, Groesch TD, Kuhn RJ, Post CB (2004) Solution structure of dengue virus capsid protein reveals another fold. Proc. Natl. Acad. Sci. USA 101(10):3414-9.

[13] Zhang Y, Corver J, Chipman PR, Zhang W, Pletnev SV, Sedlak D, et al. (2003) Structures of immature flavivirus particles. EMBO J. 22(11):2604-13.

[14] Stadler K, Allison SL, Schalich J, Heinz FX (1997) Proteolytic activation of tick-borne encephalitis virus by furin. J. Virol. 71(11):8475-81.

[15] Kuhn RJ, Zhang W, Rossmann MG, Pletnev SV, Corver J, Lenches E, et al. (2002) Structure of Dengue virus: Implications for flavivirus organization, maturation, and fusion. Cell 108(5):717-25.

[16] Mukhopadhyay S, Kuhn RJ, Rossmann MG (2005) A structural perspective of the flavivirus life cycle. Nat. Rev. Microbiol. 3(1):13-22.

[17] Nelson S, Jost CA, Xu Q, Ess J, Martin JE, Oliphant T, et al. (2008) Maturation of West Nile virus modulates sensitivity to antibody-mediated neutralization. PLoS Pathog. 4(5).

[18] Nybakken GE, Nelson CA, Chen BR, Diamond MS, Fremont DH (2006). Crystal structure of the West Nile virus envelope glycoprotein. J. Virol. 80(23):11467-74.

[19] Macdonald J, Tonry J, Hall RA, Williams B, Palacios G, Ashok MS, et al. (2005) NS1 protein secretion during the acute phase of West Nile virus infection. J. Virol. 79(22):13924-33.

[20] Chang HH, Shyu HF, Wang YM, Sun DS, Shyu RH, Tang SS, et al. (2002) Facilitation of cell adhesion by immobilized dengue viral nonstructural protein 1 (NS1): arginine-glycine-aspartic acid structural mimicry within the dengue viral NS1 antigen. J. Infect. Dis. 186(6):743-51.

[21] Young PR, Hilditch PA, Bletchly C, Halloran W (2000) An antigen capture enzyme-linked immunosorbent assay reveals high levels of the dengue virus protein NS1 in the sera of infected patients. J. Clin. Microbiol. 38(3):1053-7.

[22] Lin CF, Lei HY, Shiau AL, Liu CC, Liu HS, Yeh TM, et al. (2003) Antibodies from dengue patient sera cross-react with endothelial cells and induce damage. J. Med. Virol. 69(1):82-90.

[23] Chung KM, Liszewski MK, Nybakken G, Davis AE, Townsend RR, Fremont DH, et al. (2006) West Nile virus nonstructural protein NS1 inhibits complement activation by binding the regulatory protein factor H. Proc. Natl. Acad. Sci. USA 103(50):19111-6.

[24] Mackenzie JM, Khromykh AA, Jones MK, Westaway EG (1998). Subcellular localization and some biochemical properties of the flavivirus Kunjin nonstructural proteins NS2A and NS4A. Virology 245(2):203-15.

[25] Kummerer BM, Rice CM (2002) Mutations in the yellow fever virus nonstructural protein NS2A selectively block production of infectious particles. J. Virol. 76(10):4773-84.

[26] Liu WJ, Chen HB, Khromykh AA (2003) Molecular and functional analyses of Kunjin virus infectious cDNA clones demonstrate the essential roles for NS2A in virus assembly and for a nonconservative residue in NS3 in RNA replication. J. Virol. 77(14):7804-13.

[27] Liu WJ, Wang XJ, Clark DC, Lobigs M, Hall RA, Khromykh AA (2006) A single amino acid substitution in the West Nile virus nonstructural protein NS2A disables its ability to inhibit alpha/beta interferon induction and attenuates virus virulence in mice. J. Virol. 80(5):2396-404.

[28] Chambers TJ, Weir RC, Grakoui A, McCourt DW, Bazan JF, Fletterick RJ, et al. (1990) Evidence that the N-terminal domain of nonstructural protein NS3 from yellow fever virus is a serine protease responsible for site-specific cleavages in the viral polyprotein. Proceedings of the National Academy of Sciences 87(22):8898-902.

[29] Gorbalenya AE, Donchenko AP, Koonin EV, Blinov VM (1989) N-terminal domains of putative helicases of flavi- and pestiviruses may be serine proteases. Nucleic Acids Research 17(10):3889-97.

[30] Wengler G (1991) The carboxy-terminal part of the NS 3 protein of the West Nile flavivirus can be isolated as a soluble protein after proteolytic cleavage and represents an RNA-stimulated NTPase. Virology 184(2):707-15.

[31] Chappell KJ, Stoermer MJ, Fairlie DP, Young PR (2008) Mutagenesis of the West Nile virus NS2B cofactor domain reveals two regions essential for protease activity. Journal of General Virology 89(4):1010-4.

[32] Robin G, Chappell K, Stoermer MJ, Hu S-H, Young PR, Fairlie DP, et al. (2009) Structure of West Nile Vvirus NS3 protease: Ligand stabilization of the catalytic conformation. J. Mol. Biol. 385(5):1568-77.

[33] Gorbalenya AE, Koonin EV, Donchenko AP, Blinov VM. (1989) Two related superfamilies of putative helicases involved in replication, recombination, repair and expression of DNA and RNA genomes. Nucleic Acids Res. 17(12):4713-30

[34] Wengler G (1993) The NS 3 nonstructural protein of flaviviruses contains an RNA triphosphatase activity. Virology 197(1):265-73.

[35] Warrener P, Tamura JK, Collett MS (1993) RNA-stimulated NTPase activity associated with yellow fever virus NS3 protein expressed in bacteria. J. Virol. 67(2):989-96.

[36] Li H, Clum S, You S, Ebner KE, Padmanabhan R (1999) The serine protease and RNA-stimulated nucleoside triphosphatase and RNA helicase functional domains of dengue virus type 2 NS3 converge within a region of 20 amino acids. J. Virol. 73(4):3108-16.

[37] Luo D, Xu T, Watson RP, Scherer-Becker D, Sampath A, Jahnke W, et al. (2008) Insights into RNA unwinding and ATP hydrolysis by the flavivirus NS3 protein. EMBO J. 27(23):3209-19.

[38] Frick DN, Banik S, Rypma RS (2007) Role of divalent metal cations in ATP hydrolysis catalyzed by the hepatitis C virus NS3 helicase: magnesium provides a bridge for ATP to fuel unwinding. J. Mol. Biol. 365(4):1017-32.

[39] Lin C, Amberg SM, Chambers TJ, Rice CM (1993) Cleavage at a novel site in the NS4A region by the yellow fever virus NS2B-3 proteinase is a prerequisite for processing at the downstream 4A/4B signalase site. J Virol 67(4):2327-35.

[40] Miller S, Kastner S, Krijnse-Locker J, Bühler S, Bartenschlager R (2007) The non-structural protein 4A of Dengue virus is an integral membrane protein inducing membrane alterations in a 2K-regulated manner. Journal of Biological Chemistry 282(12):8873-82.

[41] Shiryaev SA, Chernov AV, Aleshin AE, Shiryaeva TN, Strongin AY (2009). NS4A regulates the ATPase activity of the NS3 helicase: a novel cofactor role of the non-structural protein NS4A from West Nile virus. J. Gen. Virol. 90(Pt 9):2081-5.

[42] Miller S, Sparacio S, Bartenschlager R Subcellular localization and membrane topology of the Dengue virus type 2 Non-structural protein 4B. J. Biol. Chem. (2006) 281(13):8854-63.

[43] Umareddy I, Chao A, Sampath A, Gu F, Vasudevan SG (2006) Dengue virus NS4B interacts with NS3 and dissociates it from single-stranded RNA. J. Gen. Virol. 87(Pt 9):2605-14.

[44] Guo J-T, Hayashi J, Seeger C (2005) West Nile virus inhibits the signal transduction pathway of alpha interferon. J. Virol. 79(3):1343-50.

[45] Liu WJ, Wang XJ, Mokhonov VV, Shi PY, Randall R, Khromykh AA (2005) Inhibition of interferon signaling by the New York 99 strain and Kunjin subtype of West Nile virus involves blockage of STAT1 and STAT2 activation by nonstructural proteins. J. Virol. 79(3):1934-42.

[46] Muñoz-Jordán JL, Sánchez-Burgos GG, Laurent-Rolle M, García-Sastre A (2003) Inhibition of interferon signaling by dengue virus. Proceedings of the National Academy of Sciences 100(24):14333-8.

[47] Bisaillon M, Lemay G (1997) Viral and Cellular Enzymes Involved in Synthesis of mRNA Cap Structure. Virology 236(1):1-7.

[48] Egloff MP, Benarroch D, Selisko B, Romette JL, Canard B (2002) An RNA cap (nucleoside-2'-O-)-methyltransferase in the flavivirus RNA polymerase NS5: crystal structure and functional characterization. EMBO J. 21(11):2757-68.

[49] Davidson AD (2009) Chapter 2 new insights into flavivirus nonstructural protein 5. In: Karl Maramorosch AJS, Frederick AM, editors. Advances in Virus Research: Academic Press Volume 74 p. 41-101.

[50] Smit JM, Moesker B, Rodenhuis-Zybert I, Wilschut J (2011). Flavivirus cell entry and membrane fusion. Viruses 3(2):160-71.

[51] Davis CW, Nguyen H-Y, Hanna SL, Sánchez MD, Doms RW, Pierson TC (2006) West Nile virus discriminates between DC-SIGN and DC-SIGNR for cellular attachment and infection. J. Virol. 80(3):1290-301.

[52] Chu JJ-h, Ng M-L (2004). Interaction of West Nile virus with $\alpha v\beta 3$ integrin mediates virus entry into cells. Journal of Biological Chemistry 279(52):54533-41.

[53] Medigeshi GR, Hirsch AJ, Streblow DN, Nikolich-Zugich J, Nelson JA (2008) West Nile virus entry requires cholesterol-rich membrane microdomains and is independent of alphavbeta3 integrin. J. Virol. 82(11):5212-9.

[54] Krishnan MN, Sukumaran B, Pal U, Agaisse H, Murray JL, Hodge TW, et al. (2007) Rab 5 is required for the cellular entry of Dengue and West Nile Viruses. J Virol.

[55] Thepparit C, Smith DR (2004) Serotype-specific entry of dengue virus into liver cells: identification of the 37-kilodalton/67-kilodalton high-affinity laminin receptor as a dengue virus serotype 1 receptor. J. Virol. 78(22):12647-56.

[56] Bogachek MV, Protopopova EV, Loktev VB, Zaitsev BN, Favre M, Sekatskii SK, et al. (2008) Immunochemical and single molecule force spectroscopy studies of specific interaction between the laminin binding protein and the West Nile virus surface glycoprotein E domain II. Journal of Molecular Recognition 21(1):55-62.

[57] Chen YC, Wang SY, King CC (1999) Bacterial lipopolysaccharide inhibits dengue virus infection of primary human monocytes/macrophages by blockade of virus entry via a CD14-dependent mechanism. J. Virol. 73(4):2650-7.

[58] Jindadamrongwech S, Thepparit C, Smith DR (2004) Identification of GRP 78 (BiP) as a liver cell expressed receptor element for dengue virus serotype 2. Archives of Virology 149(5):915-27.

[59] Reyes-del Valle J, Chávez-Salinas S, Medina F, del Angel RM (2005) Heat shock protein 90 and heat shock protein 70 are components of dengue virus receptor complex in human cells. J Virol;79(8):4557-67.

[60] Lee JW-M, Chu JJ-H, Ng M-L(2006) Quantifying the specific binding between West Nile virus envelope domain III protein and the cellular receptor $\alpha v\beta 3$ integrin. Journal of Biological Chemistry 281(3):1352-60.

[61] Chu JJH, Ng ML (2004). Infectious entry of West Nile virus occurs through a clathrin-mediated endocytic pathway. J. Virol. 78(19):10543-55.

[62] Nawa M, Takasaki T, Yamada K, Kurane I, Akatsuka T (2003). Interference in Japanese encephalitis virus infection of Vero cells by a cationic amphiphilic drug, chlorpromazine. J. Gen. Virol. 84(Pt 7):1737-41.

[63] Chu JJH, Leong PWH, Ng ML (2006) Analysis of the endocytic pathway mediating the infectious entry of mosquito-borne flavivirus West Nile into Aedes albopictus mosquito (C6/36) cells. Virology 349(2):463-75.

[64] Liao M, Martín CS-S, Zheng A, Kielian M (2010) In vitro reconstitution reveals key intermediate states of trimer formation by the dengue virus membrane fusion protein. J. Virol. 84(11):5730-40.
[65] Cleaves GR, Ryan TE, Schlesinger RW (1981) Identification and characterization of type 2 dengue virus replicative intermediate and replicative form RNAs. Virology 111(1):73-83.
[66] Chu PW, Westaway EG (1987) Characterization of Kunjin virus RNA-dependent RNA polymerase: reinitiation of synthesis in vitro. Virology 157(2):330-7.
[67] Konishi E, Mason PW (1993) Proper maturation of the Japanese encephalitis virus envelope glycoprotein requires cosynthesis with the premembrane protein. J. Virol. 67(3):1672-5.
[68] Wengler G (1989) Cell-associated West Nile flavivirus is covered with E+pre-M protein heterodimers which are destroyed and reorganized by proteolytic cleavage during virus release. J. Virol. 63(6):2521-6.
[69] Moesker B, Rodenhuis-Zybert IA, Meijerhof T, Wilschut J, Smit JM (2010) Characterization of the functional requirements of West Nile virus membrane fusion. Journal of General Virology 91(2):389-93.
[70] Dejnirattisai W, Jumnainsong A, Onsirisakul N, Fitton P, Vasanawathana S, Limpitikul W, et al. (2010) Cross-reacting antibodies enhance dengue virus infection in humans. Science 328(5979):745-8.
[71] Rodenhuis-Zybert IA, van der Schaar HM, da Silva Voorham JM, van der Ende-Metselaar H, Lei HY, Wilschut J, et al. (2010) Immature dengue virus: a veiled pathogen? PLoS Pathog 6(1):e1000718.
[72] Plevka P, Battisti AJ, Junjhon J, Winkler DC, Holdaway HA, Keelapang P, et al. (2011) Maturation of flaviviruses starts from one or more icosahedrally independent nucleation centres. EMBO Rep. 12(6):602-6.
[73] Work TH, Hurlbut HS, Taylor RM (1955) Indigenous wild birds of the Nile Delta as potential West Nile virus circulating reservoirs. Am. J. Trop. Med. Hyg. 4(5):872-88.
[74] The CDC Database [homepage on the internet] USA, CDC, Division of Vector-Borne Diseases [updated 2009 April 28; cited 2012 Apr 8]. Available from: http://www.cdc.gov/ncidod/dvbid/westnile/birds&mammals.htm
[75] Charatan F (2002) Organ transplants and blood transfusions may transmit West Nile virus. BMJ. 325:566.
[76] Alpert SG, Fergerson J, Noel LP (2003) Intrauterine West Nile virus: ocular and systemic findings.Am J Ophthalmol. 136:733–735.
[77] Centers for Disease Control and Prevention (2002) Possible West Nile virus transmission to an infant through breast-feeding. Michigan JAMA. 288:1976–1977.
[78] Mostashari F, Bunning ML, Kitsutani PT, Singer DA, Nash D, Cooper MJ, et al. (2001) Epidemic West Nile encephalitis, New York, 1999: results of a household-based seroepidemiological survey. Lancet 358(9278):261-4.
[79] Lim SM, Koraka P, Osterhaus AD, Martina BE (2011) West Nile virus: immunity and pathogenesis. Viruses 3(6):811-28.

[80] Bunning ML, Bowen RA, Cropp CB, Sullivan KG, Davis BS, Komar N, et al. (2002) Experimental infection of horses with West Nile virus. Emerg. Infect. Dis. 8(4):380-6.

[81] Komar N, Langevin S, Hinten S, Nemeth N, Edwards E, Hettler D, et al. (2003) Experimental infection of North American birds with the New York 1999 strain of West Nile virus. Emerg. Infect. Dis. 9(3):311-22.

[82] Rappole JH, Derrickson SR, Hubalek Z (2000) Migratory birds and spread of West Nile virus in the Western Hemisphere. Emerg. Infect. Dis. 6(4):319-28.

[83] Komar O, Robbins MB, Contreras GG, Benz BW, Klenk K, Blitvich BJ, et al. (2005) West Nile virus survey of birds and mosquitoes in the Dominican Republic. Vector Borne Zoonotic Dis. 5(2):120-6.

[84] Calistri P, Giovannini A, Hubalek Z, Ionescu A, Monaco F, Savini G, et al. (2010) Epidemiology of west nile in europe and in the mediterranean basin. Open Virol. J. 4:29-37.

[85] Ernek E, Kozuch O, Nosek J, Teplan J, Folk C (1977) Arboviruses in birds captured in Slovakia. J. Hyg. Epidemiol. Microbiol. Immunol. 21(3):353-9.

[86] Jourdain E, Olsen B, Lundkvist A, Hubalek Z, Sikutova S, Waldenstrom J, et al. (2011) Surveillance for West Nile virus in wild birds from northern Europe. Vector Borne Zoonotic Dis. 11(1):77-9.

[87] Valiakos G, Touloudi A, Athanasiou L, Giannakopoulos A, Iacovakis C, Birtsas P, et al. (2011) Exposure of Eurasian magpies and turtle doves to West Nile virus during a major human outbreak, Greece, 2011. European Journal of Wildlife Research: DOI:10.1007/s10344-011-0603-1.

[88] Mackenzie JS, Williams DT (2009) The zoonotic flaviviruses of southern, south-eastern and eastern Asia, and Australasia: the potential for emergent viruses. Zoonoses Public Health 56(6-7):338-56.

[89] May FJ, Davis CT, Tesh RB, Barrett ADT (2011) Phylogeography of West Nile virus: from the cradle of evolution in Africa to Eurasia, Australia, and the Americas. J. Virol. 85(6):2964-74.

[90] Bondre VP, Jadi RS, Mishra AC, Yergolkar PN, Arankalle VA (2007) West Nile virus isolates from India: evidence for a distinct genetic lineage. J. Gen. Virol. 88(Pt 3):875-84.

[91] Bakonyi T, Hubalek Z, Rudolf I, Nowotny N (2005) Novel flavivirus or new lineage of West Nile virus, central Europe. Emerg. Infect. Dis. 11(2):225-31.

[92] Lvov DK, Butenko AM, Gromashevsky VL, Kovtunov AI, Prilipov AG, Kinney R, et al. (2004) West Nile virus and other zoonotic viruses in Russia: examples of emerging-reemerging situations. Arch. Virol. Suppl. (18):85-96.

[93] Vazquez A, Sanchez-Seco MP, Ruiz S, Molero F, Hernandez L, Moreno J, et al. (2010) Putative new lineage of west nile virus, Spain. Emerg. Infect. Dis. 16(3):549-52.

[94] Bakonyi T, Ivanics E, Erdelyi K, Ursu K, Ferenczi E, Weissenbock H, et al. (2006) Lineage 1 and 2 strains of encephalitic West Nile virus, central Europe. Emerg. Infect. Dis. 12(4):618-23.

[95] Platonov AE, Fedorova MV, Karan LS, Shopenskaya TA, Platonova OV, Zhuravlev VI (2008) Epidemiology of West Nile infection in Volgograd, Russia, in relation to climate change and mosquito (Diptera: Culicidae) bionomics. Parasitol. Res. 103 Suppl 1:S45-53.

[96] Sirbu A, Ceianu CS, Panculescu-Gatej RI, Vazquez A, Tenorio A, Rebreanu R, et al. (2011) Outbreak of West Nile virus infection in humans, Romania, July to October 2010. Euro Surveill. 16(2).
[97] Bagnarelli P, Marinelli K, Trotta D, Monachetti A, Tavio M, Del Gobbo R, et al. (2011) Human case of autochthonous West Nile virus lineage 2 infection in Italy, September 2011. Euro Surveill. 16(43).
[98] Savini G, Capelli G, Monaco F, Polci A, Russo F, Di Gennaro A, et al. (2012) Evidence of West Nile virus lineage 2 circulation in northern Italy. Vet. Microbiol. DOI:10.1016/j.vetmic.2012.02.018.
[99] Brault AC, Huang CYH, Langevin SA, Kinney RM, Bowen RA, Ramey WN, et al. (2007) A single positively selected West Nile viral mutation confers increased virogenesis in American crows. Nat. Genet. 39(9):1162-6.
[100] Lim P-Y, Behr MJ, Chadwick CM, Shi P-Y, Bernard KA (2011) Keratinocytes are cell targets of west nile virus in vivo. J. Virol. 85(10):5197-201.
[101] Byrne SN, Halliday GM, Johnston LJ, King NJC (2001) Interleukin-1beta but not tumor necrosis factor is involved in West Nile virus-induced Langerhans cell migration from the skin in C57BL/6 mice. 117(3):702-9.
[102] Johnston LJ, Halliday GM, King NJC (2000) Langerhans cells migrate to local lymph nodes following cutaneous infection with an arbovirus. J. Investig. Dermatol. 114(3):560-8.
[103] Rios M, Zhang MJ, Grinev A, Srinivasan K, Daniel S, Wood O, et al. (2006) Monocytes-macrophages are a potential target in human infection with West Nile virus through blood transfusion. Transfusion 46(4):659-67.
[104] Wang T, Town T, Alexopoulou L, Anderson JF, Fikrig E, Flavell RA (2004) Toll-like receptor 3 mediates West Nile virus entry into the brain causing lethal encephalitis. Nat. Med. 10(12):1366-73.
[105] Monath TP, Cropp CB, Harrison AK (1983) Mode of entry of a neurotropic arbovirus into the central nervous system. Reinvestigation of an old controversy. Lab. Invest. 48(4):399-410.
[106] Samuel MA, Wang H, Siddharthan V, Morrey JD, Diamond MS (2007) Axonal transport mediates West Nile virus entry into the central nervous system and induces acute flaccid paralysis. Proc. Natl. Acad. Sci. USA 104(43):17140-5.
[107] Garcia-Tapia D, Loiacono CM, Kleiboeker SB (2006) Replication of West Nile virus in equine peripheral blood mononuclear cells. Veterinary Immunology and Immunopathology 110(3–4):229-44.
[108] Lazear HM, Pinto AK, Vogt MR, Gale M, Diamond MS (2011) Beta Interferon Controls West Nile Virus Infection and Pathogenesis in Mice. J. Virol. 85(14):7186-94.
[109] Appler KK, Brown AN, Stewart BS, Behr MJ, Demarest VL, Wong SJ, et al. (2010) Persistence of West Nile Virus in the central nervous system and periphery of mice. PLoS ONE 5(5):e10649.
[110] Busch MP, Kleinman SH, Tobler LH, Kamel HT, Norris PJ, Walsh I, et al. (2008) Virus and antibody dynamics in acute west nile virus infection. J. Infect. Dis. 198(7):984-93.

[111] Panella NA, Kerst AJ, Lanciotti RS, Bryant P, Wolf B, Komar N (2001) Comparative West Nile virus detection in organs of naturally infected American Crows (Corvus brachyrhynchos). Emerg. Infect. Dis. 7(4):754-5.

[112] Arno W, Shivers J, Carroll L, Bender J (2004) Pathological and immunohistochemical findings in American crows (Corvus brachyrhynchos) naturally infected with West Nile virus. Journal of Veterinary Diagnostic Investigation 16(4):329-33.

[113] Owen J, Moore F, Panella N, Edwards E, Bru R, Hughes M, et al. (2006) Migrating birds as dispersal vehicles for West Nile virus. EcoHealth 3(2):79-85.

[114] Nemeth N, Young G, Ndaluka C, Bielefeldt-Ohmann H, Komar N, Bowen R. (2009) Persistent West Nile virus infection in the house sparrow (Passer domesticus). Arch. Virol. 154(5):783-9.

[115] Reisen WK, Fang Y, Lothrop HD, Martinez VM, Wilson J, Oconnor P, et al. (2006) Overwintering of West Nile virus in southern California. J. Med. Entomol. 43(2):344-55.

[116] Le Bon A, Thompson C, Kamphuis E, Durand V, Rossmann C, Kalinke U, et al. (2006) Cutting edge: enhancement of antibody responses through direct stimulation of B and T cells by type I IFN. The Journal of Immunology 176(4):2074-8.

[117] Marrack P, Kappler J, Mitchell T (1999) Type I Interferons keep activated T Cells alive. J. Exp. Med. 189(3):521-30.

[118] Asselin-Paturel C, Brizard G, Chemin K, Boonstra A, O'Garra A, Vicari A, et al. (2005) Type I interferon dependence of plasmacytoid dendritic cell activation and migration. J. Exp. Med. 201(7):1157-67.

[119] Chesler DA, Reiss CS (2002) The role of IFN-γ in immune responses to viral infections of the central nervous system. Cytokine Growth Factor Reviews 13(6):441-54.

[120] Schroder K, Hertzog PJ, Ravasi T, Hume DA (2004) Interferon-γ: an overview of signals, mechanisms and functions. Journal of Leukocyte Biology 75(2):163-89.

[121] Diamond MS (2009) Virus and host determinants of West Nile virus pathogenesis. PLoS Pathog 5(6):e1000452.

[122] Chan-Tack KM, Forrest G (2005) Failure of interferon alpha-2b in a patient with West Nile virus meningoencephalitis and acute flaccid paralysis. Scandinavian Journal of Infectious Diseases 37(11-12):944-6.

[123] Barton GM, Medzhitov R (2003) Linking Toll-like receptors to IFN-alpha/beta expression. Nat Immunol 4(5):432-3.

[124] Keller BC, Fredericksen BL, Samuel MA, Mock RE, Mason PW, Diamond MS, et al. (2006) Resistance to Alpha/Beta Interferon is a determinant of West Nile virus replication fitness and virulence. J. Virol. 80(19):9424-34.

[125] Yoneyama M, Kikuchi M, Matsumoto K, Imaizumi T, Miyagishi M, Taira K, et al. (2005) Shared and unique functions of the DExD/H-Box helicases RIG-I, MDA5, and LGP2 in Antiviral Innate Immunity. The Journal of Immunology 175(5):2851-8.

[126] Yoneyama M, Kikuchi M, Natsukawa T, Shinobu N, Imaizumi T, Miyagishi M, et al. (2004) The RNA helicase RIG-I has an essential function in double-stranded RNA-induced innate antiviral responses. Nat. Immunol. 5(7):730-7.

[127] Roozendaal R, Carroll MC (2006) Emerging Patterns in Complement-Mediated Pathogen Recognition. Cell 125(1):29-32.

[128] Mehlhop E, Diamond MS (2006) Protective immune responses against West Nile virus are primed by distinct complement activation pathways. J. Exp. Med. 203(5):1371-81.

[129] Mehlhop E, Whitby K, Oliphant T, Marri A, Engle M, Diamond MS (2005) Complement activation is required for induction of a protective antibody response against West Nile virus infection. J. Virol. 79(12):7466-77.

[130] Ben-Nathan D, Huitinga I, Lustig S, van Rooijen N, Kobiler D (1996) West Nile virus neuroinvasion and encephalitis induced by macrophage depletion in mice. Arch. Virol. 141(3-4):459-69.

[131] Wang T, Gao Y, Scully E, Davis CT, Anderson JF, Welte T, et al. (2006) γδ T Cells facilitate adaptive immunity against West Nile virus infection in mice. The Journal of Immunology 177(3):1825-32.

[132] Diamond MS, Shrestha B, Marri A, Mahan D, Engle M (2003) B Cells and Antibody play critical roles in the immediate defense of disseminated infection by West Nile encephalitis virus. J. Virol. 77(4):2578-86.

[133] Diamond MS, Sitati EM, Friend LD, Higgs S, Shrestha B, Engle M (2003) A critical role for induced IgM in the protection against West Nile virus infection. J. Exp. Med. 198(12):1853-62.

[134] Shrestha B, Diamond MS (2004) Role of CD8+ T Cells in control of West Nile virus infection. J. Virol. 78(15):8312-21.

[135] Gollins SW, Porterfield JS (1986) A new mechanism for the neutralization of enveloped viruses by antiviral antibody. Nature 321(6067):244-6.

[136] Nybakken GE, Oliphant T, Johnson S, Burke S, Diamond MS, Fremont DH (2005) Structural basis of West Nile virus neutralization by a therapeutic antibody. Nature 437(7059):764-9.

[137] Roehrig JT (2003) Antigenic structure of flavivirus proteins. Adv. Virus Res. 59:141-75.

[138] Pincus S, Mason PW, Konishi E, Fonseca BA, Shope RE, Rice CM, et al. (1992) Recombinant vaccinia virus producing the prM and E proteins of yellow fever virus protects mice from lethal yellow fever encephalitis. Virology 187(1):290-7.

[139] Pierson TC, Fremont DH, Kuhn RJ, Diamond MS (2008) Structural insights into the mechanisms of antibody-mediated neutralization of flavivirus infection: implications for vaccine development. Cell Host Microbe 4(3):229-38.

[140] Della-Porta AJ, Westaway EG (1978) A Multi-Hit model for the neutralization of animal viruses. Journal of General Virology 38(1):1-19.

[141] Pierson TC, Xu Q, Nelson S, Oliphant T, Nybakken GE, Fremont Daved H, et al. (2007) The stoichiometry of antibody-mediated neutralization and enhancement of West Nile virus infection. Cell Host Microbe 1(2):135-45.

[142] Klasse PJ, Burton DR (2007) Antibodies to West Nile virus: A double-edged sword. Cell Host Microbe 1(2):87-9.

[143] Chung KM, Nybakken GE, Thompson BS, Engle MJ, Marri A, Fremont DH, et al. (2006) Antibodies against West Nile virus nonstructural protein NS1 prevent lethal infection through Fc γ Receptor-dependent and independent mechanisms. J. Virol. 80(3):1340-51.

[144] Harty JT, Badovinac VP (2002) Influence of effector molecules on the CD8+ T cell response to infection. Curr. Opin. Immunol. 14(3):360-5.

[145] Russell JH, Ley TJ. (2002) Lymphocyte-mediated cytotoxicity. Annu. Rev. Immunol. 20:323-70.

[146] Shrestha B, Samuel MA, Diamond MS (2006) CD8+ T Cells require perforin to clear West Nile virus from infected neurons. J. Virol. 80(1):119-29.

[147] Wang Y, Lobigs M, Lee E, Mullbacher A (2004) Exocytosis and Fas mediated cytolytic mechanisms exert protection from West Nile virus induced encephalitis in mice. Immunol. Cell Biol. 82(2):170-3.

[148] Sitati EM, Diamond MS (2006) CD4+ T-Cell responses are required for clearance of West Nile virus from the Central Nervous System. J. Virol. 80(24):12060-9.

[149] Shrestha B, Gottlieb D, Diamond MS (2003) Infection and injury of neurons by West Nile encephalitis virus. J. Virol. 77(24):13203-13.

[150] Wang Y, Lobigs M, Lee E, Müllbacher A (2003) CD8+ T Cells mediate recovery and immunopathology in West Nile virus encephalitis. J. Virol. 77(24):13323-34.

[151] Klein RS, Lin E, Zhang B, Luster AD, Tollett J, Samuel MA, et al. (2005) Neuronal CXCL10 directs CD8+ T-Cell recruitment and control of West Nile virus encephalitis. J. Virol. 79(17):11457-66.

[152] Glass WG, Lim JK, Cholera R, Pletnev AG, Gao J-L, Murphy PM (2005) Chemokine receptor CCR5 promotes leukocyte trafficking to the brain and survival in West Nile virus infection. J. Exp. Med. 202(8):1087-98.

[153] Beasley DWC, Whiteman MC, Zhang S, Huang CY-H, Schneider BS, Smith DR, et al. (2005) Envelope protein glycosylation status influences mouse neuroinvasion phenotype of genetic lineage 1 West Nile virus strains. J. Virol. 79(13):8339-47.

[154] Kasturi L, Eshleman JR, Wunner WH, Shakin-Eshleman SH (1995) The hydroxy amino acid in an Asn-X-Ser/Thr sequon can influence N-linked core glycosylation efficiency and the level of expression of a cell surface glycoprotein. J. Biol. Chem. 270(24):14756-61.

[155] Modis Y, Ogata S, Clements D, Harrison SC (2003) A ligand-binding pocket in the dengue virus envelope glycoprotein. Proceedings of the National Academy of Sciences 100(12):6986-91.

[156] Rey FA, Heinz FX, Mandl C, Kunz C, Harrison SC (1995) The envelope glycoprotein from tick-borne encephalitis virus at 2Å resolution. Nature 375(6529):291-8.

[157] Murata R, Eshita Y, Maeda A, Maeda J, Akita S, Tanaka T, et al. (2010) Glycosylation of the West Nile Virus Envelope Protein Increases In Vivo and In Vitro Viral Multiplication in Birds. Am J Trop Med Hyg 82(4):696-704.

[158] Papa A, Bakonyi T, Xanthopoulou K, Vazquez A, Tenorio A, Nowotny N. (2011) Genetic characterization of West Nile virus lineage 2, Greece, 2010. Emerg. Infect. Dis. 17(5):920-2.

[159] Wicker JA, Whiteman MC, Beasley DWC, Davis CT, Zhang S, Schneider BS, et al. (2006) A single amino acid substitution in the central portion of the West Nile virus NS4B protein confers a highly attenuated phenotype in mice. Virology 349(2):245-53.

[160] Muñoz-Jordán JL, Laurent-Rolle M, Ashour J, Martínez-Sobrido L, Ashok M, Lipkin WI, et al. (2005) Inhibition of Alpha/Beta Interferon Signaling by the NS4B Protein of Flaviviruses. J. Virol. 79(13):8004-13.

[161] Puig-Basagoiti F, Tilgner M, Bennett CJ, Zhou Y, Muñoz-Jordán JL, García-Sastre A, et al. (2007) A mouse cell-adapted NS4B mutation attenuates West Nile virus RNA synthesis. Virology 361(1):229-41.

[162] Welte T, Xie G, Wicker JA, Whiteman MC, Li L, Rachamallu A, et al. (2011) Immune responses to an attenuated West Nile virus NS4B-P38G mutant strain. Vaccine 29(29–30):4853-61.

[163] Rossi SL, Fayzulin R, Dewsbury N, Bourne N, Mason PW (2007) Mutations in West Nile virus nonstructural proteins that facilitate replicon persistence in vitro attenuate virus replication in vitro and in vivo. Virology 364(1):184-95.

[164] Chaskopoulou A, Dovas C, Chaintoutis S, Bouzalas I, Ara G, Papanastassopoulou M. (2011) Evidence of enzootic circulation of West Nile virus (Nea Santa-Greece-2010, lineage 2), Greece, May to July 2011. Euro Surveill. 16(31).

[165] Sotelo E, Fernandez-Pinero J, Llorente F, Aguero M, Hoefle U, Blanco JM, et al. (2009) Characterization of West Nile virus isolates from Spain: new insights into the distinct West Nile virus eco-epidemiology in the Western Mediterranean. Virology 395(2):289-97.

[166] Sotelo E, Gutierrez-Guzman AV, Del Amo J, Llorente F, El-Harrak M, Perez-Ramirez E, et al. (2011) Pathogenicity of two recent Western Mediterranean West Nile virus isolates in a wild bird species indigenous to Southern Europe: the red-legged partridge. Vet. Res. 42(1):11.

[167] Mertens E, Kajaste-Rudnitski A, Torres S, Funk A, Frenkiel M-P, Iteman I, et al. (2010) Viral determinants in the NS3 helicase and 2K peptide that promote West Nile virus resistance to antiviral action of 2′,5′-oligoadenylate synthetase 1b. Virology 399(1):176-85.

[168] Botha EM, Markotter W, Wolfaardt M, Paweska JT, Swanepoel R, Palacios G, et al. (2008) Genetic determinants of virulence in pathogenic lineage 2 West Nile virus strains. Emerg. Infect. Dis. 14(2):222-30.

Chapter 3

Hepatitis B Virus Genetic Diversity: Disease Pathogenesis

MariaKuttikan Jayalakshmi, Narayanan Kalyanaraman
and Ramasamy Pitchappan

Additional information is available at the end of the chapter

http://dx.doi.org/10.5772/53818

1. Introduction

Hepatitis B Virus (HBV) infection is a global health problem: an estimated two billion people (one-third of the global population) have been infected with HBV at some point in their life; of these, more than 350 million suffer from chronic HBV infection, resulting in over 600,000 deaths each year, mainly from cirrhosis or liver cancer [1]. More than 10% of the global chronic HBV population resides in India [2]; infection may lead to liver damage that results in acute or chronic hepatitis, liver cirrhosis, and hepatocellular carcinoma (HCC) (Figure 1). HBV infection was first identified in 1965 when Blumberg and co-workers [3] found the hepatitis B surface antigen (HBsAg), originally termed as *Australia antigen*. Enhanced viral replication leading to a vigorous and extensive immune response may lead to massive liver injury resulting spontaneously into fulminant hepatic failure. The seriousness of disease incidence is mainly related to various host factors (age, gender, duration of infection, immune response) and viral factors (viral load, genotype, quasispecies) (Figure 2). Recent evidence shows that considerable molecular variation occurs throughout the HBV genome, which is correlated with geographical distribution of genotypes and severity of disease.

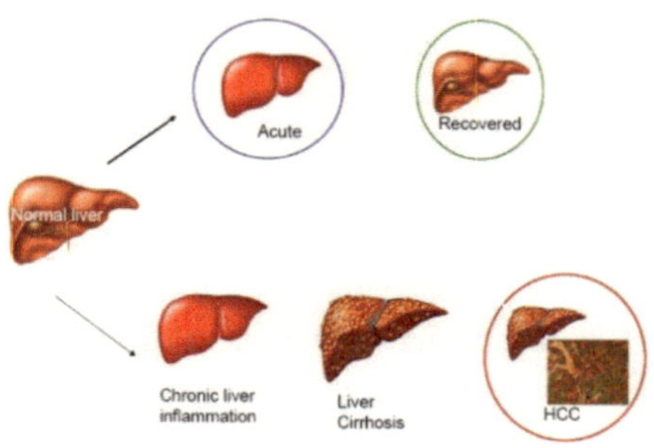

Figure 1. HBV mediated liver damage among various stages

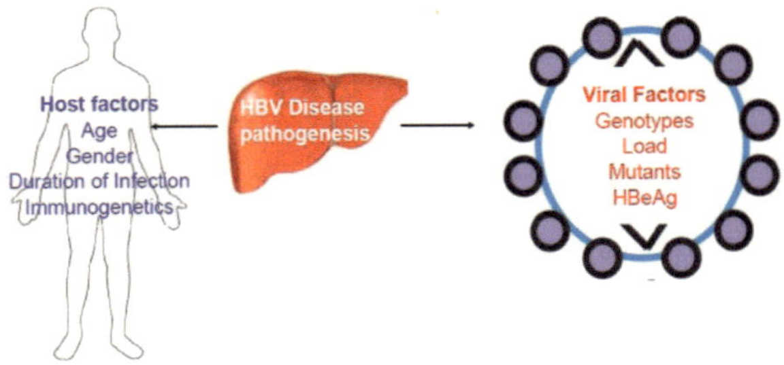

Figure 2. Host – pathogen factors in disease manifestation

1.1. HBV evolution

The history and origin of HBV is partially understood. The evolution of HBV can be traced from lowest vertebrates such as the birds infecting virus i.e. avian hepadnavirus which shares a sequence homology of 40%, non-primate such as rodents infecting wood chuck HBV viruses shares 80% homology [4, 5]. However, highest incidence of greater than 94% of homology is found to occur in primates infecting viruses suggesting an evolutionary sequence for the human HBV [6].

The long time evolution of HBV therefore leads to the occurrence of various genotypes, subgenotypes, mutants, recombinants and even quasispecies [7]. Major forces such as genetic drift, bottle neck effects, founder effects and recombination played a vital role in evolution, adaptation of HBV and become a successful pathogen in the host. The genetic variability, in conjunction with the migration of human race, has led to the divergence of HBV into genetically different groups, called genotypes, with a distinct geographic distribution. Some researchers suggest that HBV co-evolved with modern humans, as they migrated from Africa, around 100,000 years ago [8,9]. Based on the prevalence, geographic distribution and characteristic of recombinant genotypes, it can be suggested that genotypes A and D co-exist over a relatively long period, while genotypes B and C are believed to have recent epidemiological contact in Asia [10]. The genetic diversity of HBV and its geographical distribution may help us to reconstruct the evolutionary trend of HBV. This may help to generate additional genetic data on the evolution and migration pattern of man [8].

1.2. Hepatitis B Virus: Molecular virology

HBV is a hepatotropic, non-cytopathic virus and a prototype member of the family *Hepadnaviridae* with a genome size of ~3,200 base pairs. The viral genome consists of a partially double-stranded, relaxed-circular DNA (RC-DNA), comprising a complete coding strand (negative strand) and an incomplete non-coding strand (positive strand), which replicates by reverse transcription *via* an RNA intermediate. Due to reduced fidelity of the reverse transcription process, this pregenomic RNA (pgRNA) is prone to mutation. The genome encodes four overlapping reading frames that are translated to make the viral core protein (HBcAg), the surface proteins (HBsAg) , a reverse transcriptase (RT), and the hepatitis B "x" antigen (HBxAg).

1.3. Viral entry and replication

HBV has a high degree of species and tissue specificity that results in very high levels of viral replication without actually killing the infected cell directly. The mechanism through which HBV enters hepatocyte or other susceptible cells remains elusive mostly owing to lack of a proper cell culture system. As a pararetrovirus, HBV uses reverse transcription to copy its DNA genome and lack of proof-reading capability permits the emergence of mutant viral genomes and quasispecies.

Upon infecting a hepatocyte, the HBV genome is delivered in to the nuclear compartment where cellular repair enzymes are involved in repairing the viral genome into covalently closed circular DNA (cccDNA). This viral DNA acts as a transcriptional template [11, 12] for the generation of the pregenomic mRNA (pg mRNA), pre-core mRNA and all other subviral mRNAs [13, 14]. Subsequently, cccDNA is chromatinized into viral minichromosome that ultimately serves as an intrahepatic reservoir of HBV and stays throughout the life of the chronically infected host [15, 16]. The pregenomic RNA is encapsulated by the virion core particle and reversely transcribed by the viral polymerase, forming a single-strand DNA (negative strand). Subsequently, the pregenome is degraded and the negative strand DNA then acts as a template for synthesis of a positive strand DNA with variable length. Finally, the HBV genome is either encapsulated to produce virions to be secreted out, or recycled back to the nucleus to maintain a pool of cccDNA, resulting in the formation of a steady-state population of 5–50 copies of cccDNA molecules per infected hepatocyte [14, 17] (Figure 3).

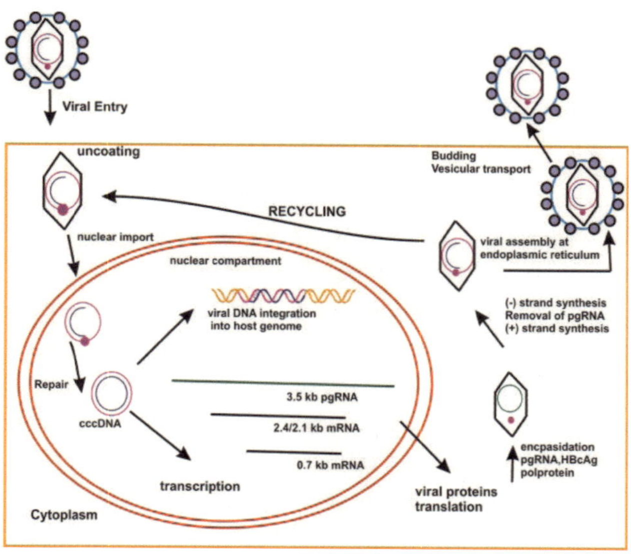

Figure 3. Viral entry and replication cycle of HBV

2. HBV genomic organization and proteins

The HBV genomes comprise a partially double-stranded 3.2kb DNA molecule, organized into 4 overlapping open-reading frames (ORFs). Four sets of mRNAs are then transcribed from the viral minichromosomes using host cell machinery, RNA polymerase II. These molecules are then transported by cellular proteins to the cytoplasm where they are translated to produce the viral proteins: hepatitis B core antigen (HBcAg or nucleocapsid protein from the 3.5 kb RNA); the soluble and secreted hepatitis B e antigen (HBeAg, from the 3.5 kb RNA); the Pol protein (from the 3.5 kb RNA, which is longer than the viral entire genome); the viral envelope proteins HBsAg (from the 2.4 and 2.0 kb RNAs) and hepatitis B X protein (HBx from the 0.7 kb RNA). The dynamic nature of individual viral proteins and insufficient immune response elicited by the infected host immune cells lead to the persistence of HBV infection

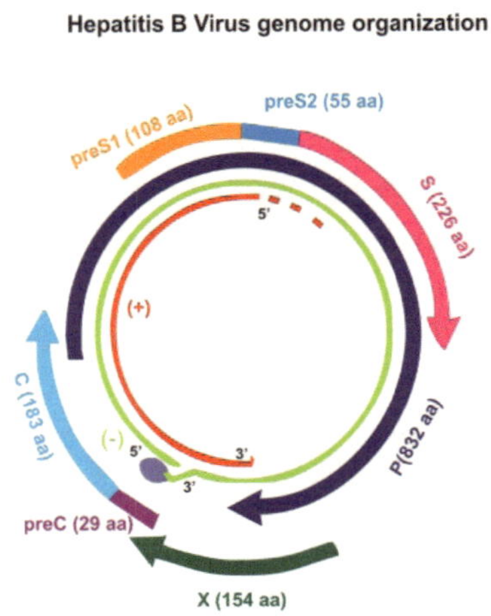

Figure 4.

2.1. Hepatitis B virus surface antigen (HBsAg)

Since Blumberg's discovery of HBsAg in 1965, it has been used as the hallmark for the diagnosis of HBV infection [18]. HBsAg is the prototype serological marker of HBV infection that characteristically appears after 1 to 10 weeks of an acute exposure to HBV but before the onset of visible symptoms or elevation of serum alanine aminotransferase (ALT) [19]. HBsAg circulates in a wide array of particulate forms such as competent virions (42 nm, Dane particles), 20 nm diameter filaments of variable length, and 20–22 nm spherical defective particles, corresponding to empty viral envelopes. It exceeds virions by a variable factor of $10^2 - 10^5$ and accumulates several hundred micrograms per ml of serum [13]. The principal function of the HBs protein as a virological structure is to enclose the viral components, in addition to playing a major role in cell membrane attachment to initiate the infection process by binding to the hepatocyte plasma membrane [20]. Persistence of HBsAg for more than 6 months indicates chronic infection and it is estimated that fewer than 5% of immunocompetent adult patients with acute hepatitis B progress to chronic infection [21]. The immune response enhancing ability of HBsAg is not clear yet it is understood that large amounts of HBsAg may induce T cell anergy, leading to decreased antibody-mediated neutralization of HBV and generalized hyporesponsiveness towards pathogens.

2.2. Hepatitis B core antigen (HBcAg)

HBcAg is the major constituent of the nucleocapsid, which is essential for viral replication. It also forms a part of ichosahedral subviral particles that packs the viral reverse polymerase and the pregenome [22] derived from the ORF-C. It has either 183 or 185 amino acids depending on the genotype of the virus. HBcAg is a particulate and multivalent protein antigen which can function as both a T cell-independent and a T cell-dependent Ag [23] and is ~1000 fold more immunogenic than the HBeAg [24]. The response of T cells to HBcAg has been reported to contribute to the resolution and seroconversion in chronic hepatitis B [25].

2.3. Hepatitis B envelope antigen (HbeAg)

HBeAg is an accessory protein of HBV, not essential for replication *in vivo* [26, 27] but important for natural infection. This antigen has been used clinically as an index of viral replication, infectivity, severity of disease, and response to treatment [28]. HBeAg may play a role in perpetuating viral infection during perinatal transmission, often resulting in chronic infection and eliciting HBe/HBcAg-specific T helper cell tolerance *in utero* [29, 30].

HBeAg is a non-particulate secretory protein discovered by Magnius and Espmark in 1972 [31]. It is derived after cleavage from a 212 amino acid precursor, precore protein that is encoded by the HBV precore gene (the pre-C sequence and C-gene). It is highly conserved evolutionarily between all *Hepadnaviridae*. As part of the core protein, it has a nucleic acid binding activity [32] required for the pregenomic RNA encapsidation, and modulation of polymerase activity for reverse transcription of pregenome [33,34].

HBeAg is found at concentrations of greater than 10μg mL^{-1} in the plasma, which can be detected even by agar-gel immunodiffusion. Secreted HBeAg has an immunoregulatory function *in utero* by establishing T cell tolerance to HBeAg and HBcAg, which may predispose neonates born to HBV-infected mothers to develop persistent HBV infection [29]. Milich et al., [35-37] further demonstrated an immunomodulatory role of HBeAg in antigen presentation and recognition by $CD4^+$ cells.

2.4. Hepatitis B X antigen (HBxAg)

HBx antigen, a 17 kDa multifunctional, non-structural protein, comprised of 154 amino acids, which is conserved across all the mammalian infecting *Hepadnaviridae*. The X gene is the smallest of the four partially overlapping ORF of the HBV genome. The biological function of HBx protein is not yet clear however this has been implicated in causing HBV associated liver cancer.

Accumulating evidences indicate that the HBV X gene is indispensable to HBV replication, propagation and integration of viral DNA into the host's genome. The expression of full-length HBx protein is dispensable for virus production *in vitro* and a critical component of the infectivity process *in vivo* [38]. HBx protein promotes virus gene expression and replication by trans-activating the virus promoters and enhancer/promoter complexes [39,

40]. In addition, HBx accumulation enhances viral replication by altering various cellular activities including aberrant expression of molecules, involved in host cell signal transduction, transcription and proliferation, leading to viral persistence and hepatocarcinogenesis [41, 42, 43].

3. HBV viral load

HBV is reported to be present in the blood of HbeAg seropositive individuals at a concentration of approximately 10^8–10^9 viral particles mL^{-1} of blood [44]. HBV DNA is present in high titers in blood and exudates of in acute as well as chronic cases. Generally, moderate viral titers are found in saliva, semen and vaginal secretions [45, 46]. The serum levels of HBV DNA largely depend on the viral genotype, and the quantity of HBeAg in serum, which determines the progression of liver cirrhosis to carcinoma.

3.1. HBV genotypes and subgenotypes

The global HBV genome diversity is influenced by both genotypic and phenotypic variability; genotypes often evolve in the absence of selective pressure but phenotypic variability often develops in the presence of selective pressure exerted by host immune system or even during certain therapeutic measures [47].

This genetic diversity of HBV has been associated with differences in clinical and virological characteristics, indicating that they may play a role in the virus–host relationship [48]. Genotypes may result from neutral evolutionary drift of the virus genome, from recombination, or as a consequence of a long-term adaptation of HBV to genetic determinants of specific host populations. Structural and functional differences between genotypes can influence the severity, course and likelihood of complications, HBeAg seroconversion and response to treatment of HBV infection and possibly the vaccination against the virus [49].

Traditionally HBV was classified into 4 subtypes or serotypes (adr, adw, ayr, and ayw) based on antigenic determinants of HBsAg [50]. In the advent of more molecular approaches, serotyping of viral strains was replaced by various genotyping methods. Galibert *et al.* [51], published the first sequence of a complete HBV genome. Later, Okamoto *et al.* [52], analyzed 18 full length genomes and divided them into four groups or genotypes, named as A to D. The ability of HBV to adapt to the host genetics as well as immunogenic environment by genetic variation, led to the evolution of eight established genotypes (A-H): [8, 53] and two putative genotypes (I and J), each corresponding to a rather well-defined geographical distribution (Table 1). HBV genotypes A and D have worldwide distribution, whereas genotypes B and C are mostly found in Asia. In India HBV genotypes A and D are common in various parts, followed by genotype C specifically in eastern part of India [54-56]. The new genotype I is a complex recombinant form of genotypes A, C, and G [57,58]. The genotype J which was positioned phylogenetically in between the human and ape genotypes and was isolated from a 88-year-old hepatitis patient living in Okinawa, Japan who had a history of residing in Borneo during the World War II [59]. In addition, countries in which multiple genotypes circulate, co-infections and recombination events may occur leading to the emergence of hybrid strains that can become the dominant subgenotype prevailing in certain geographical regions.

Genotype	Serotype	Geography distribution	Genome (base pair)	ORF differences	HBV proteins (aa) Pre S1	Pol	Core
A (A1 - A6)	adw2	Africa, Europe, USA, Australia	3221	Insertion of aa 153 and 154 in HBc	119	845	185
B (B1 - B9)	adw2, ayw1	South East Asia, China, Japan	3215		119	843	183
C (C1 - C16)	adw2, ayr, adrq-,adrq+	South East Asia, China, Korea, Japan, Polynesia, Australia	3215		119	843	183
D (D1 - D7)	ayw2,3 and 4	Mediterranean area, Middle East, East Europe, India	3182	Deletion of aa 1-11 in preS1	108	832	183
E (ND)	ayw4	West and Central Africa	3212	Deletion of aa 11 in preS1	118	842	183
F (F1 - F4)	adw4q-	South America, Central America, Alsaka, Polynesia	3215		119	843	183
G (ND)	adw2	Europe, North America (Coinfection alsmost universal, with genotype A)	3248	Insertion of 12 aa in HBc; Deletion of aa 11 in preS1	118	842	195
H (ND)	adw4	Central America, Mexico, South United States	3215		119	843	183
I (ND)	adw	Vietnam, Laos, India	3215		119	843	183
J (ND)		Japan	3182		108	832	183

ND = No subgenotypes so far identified

Table 1. Overview of HBV major genotypes and its distribution pattern

3.2. HBV Genotyping

Currently, more than 10 different methods have been developed for HBV genotyping with variable sensitivity, specificity, turnaround time and cost. These methods include restriction fragment length polymorphisms (RFLP) [60], PCR with specific primers for single genotypes [61], multiplex-PCR for many HBV genotypes [62, 63] and on hybridization technologies [64] or real time quantification and genotyping [65] or Mass spectrometry [66]. The gold standard method for HBV genotyping is a complete genome sequencing followed by phylogenetic analysis of the sequence divergence [9, 52]. Sequence and phylogenetic analysis can also be performed on individual genes, more often in envelope (S) gene. The reliability of using individual genes or limited gene sequence will depend both on the size of the sequence analyzed and the degree of sequence homology. The HBV genotype can be determined by other methods that are based on a limited number of conserved nucleotide or amino acid differences between the genotypes. Line probe assay (LiPA) may be a suitable alternative to sequencing but it is expensive when compared to other methods such as multiplex PCR, RFLP and serotyping. Based on the sensitivity, other methods such as microarrays, real time PCR, reverse dot blot, restriction fragment mass polymorphism (RFMP), invader assay are being used [67,68]. Identification of HBV genotypes will be useful to understand the source of infection, predict clinical outcome at individual level and monitoring the development of newer viral strains at population level.

3.3. Clinical implications of HBV genotyping

Mounting evidence shows that HBeAg seroconversion rates, HBcAg seroconversion, viremia levels, viral latency, immune escape, emergence of mutants, pathogenesis of liver disease, response and resistance to antiviral therapy are all depend on the HBV genotypes and subgenotypes. Individual or combinations of the above factors are responsible for the degree of clinical heterogeneity displayed by the infected persons [69, 70].

Earlier reports from India, where genotypes A, D are prevalent and patients infected with genotype D had relatively high degree of disease severity and develop HCC [56]. Patients with genotypes C and D have a lower response rate to interferon therapy than patients infected with genotypes A or B [71,72]. An Alaskan population study which compares the clinical virological properties of five genotypes has shown that the mean age seroconversion from HBeAg to anti-HBe is significantly lower among genotypes A, B, D and F, than compared to genotype C [73]. This may be due to the development of more mutations in the basal core promoter region of genotypes C and D compared to genotypes A and B. Genotype G appears defective, and usually occurs together with another genotype, which provides transcription factors necessary for replication. Viral load of the patients with genotype mixture is usually higher than that of those infected with unique genotype.

3.4. HBV mutant (Phenotypic variants)

Phenotypic variants emerge in response to selective pressure [47]. Development of HBV mutants are often related to the persistence of cccDNA and viral factors such as the existence of quasispecies, high rate of HBV replication, error prone RT-based life cycle and adaptive mutants with compensatory mutations. Host factors include compliance with antiviral therapy, immune response, enhanced hepatic inflammatory response and host genetic background. HBV quasispecies arise due to the average daily production of $>10^{11}$ virions with a error rate of $1.4\text{-}3.2 \times 10^{-5}$ nucleotide substitutions per site per year, which results in production of all possible number of different single base changes in the HBV genome [74-76]. Active replication leads to an estimated misincorporation rate of around 10^4 owing to the lack of proof-reading (3′ – 5′ exonuclease activity) [77]. The combination of a high error rate together with an increased replication rate produces as high as 10^9 mutation day^{-1} over the entire 3.2kb genome [74, 78] but, the extreme overlapping of the ORF of the HBV genome limits the possibility of all these mutations [79].

Moreover, mutations in the HBV genome seem to play a vital role in differential outcome of this infection (Table 2). Two important mutations in the HBV virus have been associated with differential outcome such as the basal core promoter (BCP) mutation and the pre-core

(PC) mutation. BCP mutation is a double substitution, A1762T, G1764A, in the basal core region of HBV. It has clearly been associated with an increased risk of HCC and cirrhosis in multiple studies, both cross-sectional and prospective [80].

HBV Genomic region	Molecular Effect	Clinical relevance
Pre-S/S	pre-S1/pre-S2 mutations S gene mutations	Vaccine escape Immune escape Diagnostic escape High risk for HCC
Pre-C/C	pre-C stop codon mutations Core promoter mutations	HBeAg negativity Viral persistence High risk for HCC Severe forms of disease
Pol	Pol gene mutations Mutations in YMDD motif	Viral latency Viral persistence Therapy escape (resistance to antivirals)
Regulatory sequences	Core promoter mutations or Hepatocyte Nuclear Factor 1(HNF1)	HBeAg negativity High viremia Severe hepatitis
X gene	Truncated X gene (8 base pair deletion at the 3' end)	Immune escape High risk for HCC

Table 2. HBV mutants and its clinical impact

4. Treatment

Antiviral medications for the management of chronic HBV infections currently available include alpha interferon (IFN-α) and three nucleoside analogs: lamivudine, adefovir and entecavir that inhibit viral nucleocapsid formation and block viral DNA synthesis by premature chain termination [81,82]. The major determinant involved in the selection of drug-resistant mutation is the fitness of the mutants and the replication space available for the spread of mutants. In chronic hepatitis B, the replication space is provided by hepatocyte turnover, which allows the loss of HBV wild-type infected cells and the generation of non-infected hepatocytes that are susceptible to new HBV mutant infections. Long-term therapy of adefovir or entecavir mediates significant reduction in cccDNA, but still fails to eliminate chronic HBV infections [83, 84].

5. Conclusion

Among all forms of viral hepatitis, HBV infection is considered as a major infectious disease due to the broad range of clinical spectrum and the progressive complications displayed by the infected individuals. Avians, rodents and human forms of the virus have been recognized for many years and infections were assumed to be highly host specific. The geographic pattern of HBV genotype distribution is not only influenced by the host and viral factors but also by socio-economical factors like migration and immigration of people, availability of vaccine and anti-viral therapeutics. The genetic diversity of HBV has been associated with clinical outcome, and response to antiviral therapy. Various forces like natural selection pressure, antiviral drug mediated pressure and error prone high replication rate are the important factors responsible for this genetic diversity. The final outcome from this infectious disease is solely determined by specific interaction between viral components and immunogenetics of the host. Understanding the influence and the role of viral genetic diversity is considered as a prerequisite to better the treatment options.

Author details

MariaKuttikan Jayalakshmi and Narayanan Kalyanaraman
Department of Immunology, School of Biological Sciences, Madurai Kamaraj University, Madurai, India

Ramasamy Pitchappan
Chettinad University, Kelampakkam, Chennai , India

6. References

[1] Hepatitis B: World Health Organization Fact Sheet; c2008[updated august 2008] Available from: http://www.who.int/mediacentre/factsheets/fs204/en/
[2] Sarin SK et al. (2001) Profile of hepatocellular carcinoma in India: an insight into the possible etiologic associations. J Gastroenterol. Hepatol. 16(6):666-73.
[3] Blumberg BS et al. (1965) A new antigen in leukemia sera. JAMA. 191, 541-6
[4] Mandart E et al. (1984) Nucleotide sequence of a cloned duck hepatitis B virus genome: comparison with woodchuck and human hepatitis B virus sequences. J Virol. 49(3):782-92.
[5] Galibert F et al. (1982) Nucleotide sequence of a cloned wood chuck hepatitis virus genome: comparison with hepatitis B virus sequence. J Virol. 41(1):51-65.
[6] MacDonald DM et al.(2000) Detection of Hepatitis B Virus Infection in Wild-Born Chimpanzees (*Pan troglodytes verus*): Phylogenetic relationship with human and other primate genotype. J. Virol. 74(9): 4253-57
[7] Lau JY and Wright TL (1993) Molecular virology and pathogenesis of hepatitis B. Lancet. 342(8883):1335-40.
[8] Norder H et al. (2004) Genetic diversity of hepatitis B virus strains derived worldwide: genotypes, subgenotypes, and HBsAg subtypes. Intervirology. 47(6):289-309.
[9] Norder H et al. (1994) Complete genomes, phylogenetic relatedness, and structural proteins of six strains of the hepatitis B virus, four of which represent two new genotypes. Virology. 198(2):489-503.
[10] Fares MA and Holmes EC (2002) A revised evolutionary history of hepatitis B virus (HBV). J Mol Evol. 54(6):807-14.
[11] Liang TJ (2009) Hepatitis B: the virus and disease.Hepatology. 49(5):13-21.

[12] Ganem D and Prince AM (2004) Hepatitis B virus infection – natural history and clinical consequences. N Engl J Med. 350(11):1118-29.

[13] Seeger C and Mason WS (2000) Hepatitis B virus biology. Microbiol Mol Biol Rev. 64(1):51-68.

[14] Tuttleman JS et al. (1986) Formation of the pool of covalently closed circular viral DNA in hepadnavirus-infected cells. Cell. 47(3):451–60.

[15] Bock CT et al. (2001) Structural organization of the hepatitis B virus minichromosome. J Mol Biol. 307(1):183-96.

[16] Zhu Y et al. (2001) Kinetics of hepadnavirus loss from the liver during inhibition of viral DNA synthesis. J Virol. 75(1):311-22.

[17] Wu TT et al. (1990) In hepatocytes infected with duck hepatitis B virus, the template for viral RNA synthesis is amplified by an intracellular pathway. Virology. 175(1):255-61.

[18] Blumberg BS et al. (1986) Hepatitis and leukemia: their relation to Australia antigen. Bull N Y Acad Med. 44(12):1566-86.

[19] Krugman S et al. (1979) Viral hepatitis, type B. Studies on natural history and prevention re-examined. N Engl J Med. 300(3):101-6.

[20] Pontisso P et al. (1989) Identification of an attachment site for human liver plasma membranes on hepatitis B virus particles. Virology. 173(2):522-30.

[21] McMahon BJ et al. (1985) Acute hepatitis B virus infection: relation of age to the clinical expression of disease and subsequent development of the carrier state. J Infect Dis. 151(4) 599–603.

[22] Crowther RA et al. (1994) Three-dimensional structure of hepatitis B virus core particles determined by electron cryomicroscopy. Cell. 77(6):943-50.

[23] Milich DR and McLachlan (1986) The nucleocapsid of hepatitis B virus is both a T-cell-independent and a T-cell-dependent antigen. Science. 234(4782):1398-1401.

[24] Milich DR et al. (1988) Comparative immunogenicity of hepatitis B virus core and E antigens. J Immunol. 141(10):3617-24.

[25] Lau GK et al. (2002) Resolution of chronic hepatitis B and anti-HBs seroconversion in humans by adoptive transfer of immunity to hepatitis B core antigen. Gastroenterology. 122(3):614-24.

[26] Chen HS et al. (1992) The precore region of an avian hepatitis B virus is not required for viral replication. J Virol. 66(9):5682-4.

[27] Chang C et al. (1987) Expression of the precore region of an avian hepatitis B virus is not required for viral replication. J Virol 61(10):3322-5.

[28] Milich D and Liang TJ (2003) Exploring the biological basis of hepatitis B e antigen in hepatitis B virus infection. Hepatology. 38(5):1075–86.

[29] Milich DR et al. (1990) Is a function of the secreted hepatitis B e antigen to induce immunologic tolerance in utero? Proc Natl Acad Sci U S A. 87(17):6599-603.

[30] Terazawa S et al. (1991) Hepatitis B virus mutants with precore-region defects in two babies with fulminant hepatitis and their mothers positive for antibody to hepatitis B e antigen. Pediatr Res. 29(1):5-9.

[31] Magnius LO and Espmark JA (1972) New specificities in Australia antigen positive sera distinct from Le Bouvier determinants. J Immunol. 109(5):1017-21.

[32] Petit MA and Pillot J (1985) HBc and HBe antigenicity and DNA binding activity of major core protein P22 in hepatitis B virus core particles isolated from human liver cells. J Virol. 53(2):543-51.

[33] Nassal M (1992) The arginine rich domain of the hepatitis B virus core protein is required for pregenome encapsidation and productive viral positive-strand DNA synthesis but not for virus assembly. J Virol. 66(7):4107-16.

[34] Hatton T et al. (1992) RNA and DNA binding activities in hepatitis B virus capsid protein: a model for their roles in viral replication. J Virol. 66(9): 5232-41.

[35] Milich DR (1999). Do T cells "see" the hepatitis B core and e antigens differently? Gastroenterology. 116(3):765-8.

[36] Milich DR et al.(1998) The secreted hepatitis B precore antigen can modulate the immune response to the nucleocapsid:a mechanism for persistence. J Immunol.160(4):2013-21.

[37] Milich DR et al. (1993) Role of T-cell tolerance in the persistence of hepatitis B virus infection. J Immunol Emphasis Tumor Immunol. 14(3):226-33.

[38] Zoulim F et al. (1994) Woodchuck hepatitis virus X protein is required for viral infection in vivo. J Virol. 68(3):2026-30.

[39] Keasler W et al. (2007) Enhancement of hepatitis B virus replication by the regulatory X protein in vitro and in vivo. J Virol. 81(6):2656-62.

[40] Tang H et al. (2006) Molecular functions and biological roles of hepatitis B virus x protein. Cancer Sci. 97(10):977-83.

[41] Muroyama R et al. (2006) Nucletoide change of codon 38 in the X gene of hepatitis B virus genotype C is associated with an increased risk of hepatocellular carcinoma. J Hepatol. 45(6):805-12.

[42] Benhenda S et al. (2009) Hepatitis B virus X protein molecular functions and its role in virus life cycle and pathogenesis. Adv Cancer Res. 103:75-109.

[43] Murakami S (2001) Hepatitis B virus x protein: a multifunctional viral regulator. J Gastroenterol. 36(10):651-60.

[44] Dane DS et al. (1970) Virus-like particles in serum of patients with Australia-antigen-associated hepatitis. Lancet. 1(7649):695-8.

[45] Kidd- Ljunggren K et al. (2006) High levels of hepatitis B virus DNA in body fluids from chronic carriers. J Hosp Infect. 64(4): 352-7.

[46] Qian WP et al. (2005) Rapid quantification of semen hepatitis B virus DNA by realtime polymerase chain reaction. World J Gastroenterol. 11(34):5358-9.

[47] Kay A and Zoulim F (2007) Hepatitis B virus genetic variability and evolution. Virus Res. 127(2):164-76.

[48] Araujo NM et al. (2011) Hepatitis B virus infection from an evolutionary point of view: How viral, host, and environmental factors shape genotypes and subgenotypes. Infect Genet Evol. 11(6):1199-207.

[49] Chu CJ and Lok ASF (2002) Clinical significance of hepatitis B virus genotypes. Hepatology. 35(5):1274-6.

[50] Le Bouvier et al. (1972) Subtypes of Australia antigen and hepatitis-B virus. JAMA. 222(8):928-30.

[51] Galibert et al. (1979) Nucleotide sequence of the hepatitis B virus genome (subtype ayw) cloned in *E. coli*. Nature. 281(5733):646-50.

[52] Okamato et al. (1988) Typing hepatitis B virus by homology in nucleotide sequence: comparison of surface antigen subtypes. J Gen Virol. 69:2575-83.

[53] Kramvis et al. (2008) Relationship of serological subtype, basic core promoter and precore mutations to genotypes/subgenotypes of hepatitis B virus. J Med Virol. 80(1):27-46.

[54] Vivekanandan et al. (2004) Distribution of hepatitis B virus genotypes in blood donors and chronically infected patients in a tertiary care hospital in Southern India. Clin Infect Dis. 38(9):81-6.

[55] Gandhe et al.(2003). Hepatitis B virus genotypes and serotypes in Western India: lack of clinical significance. J Med Virol. 69(3):324-30.

[56] Thakur V et al. (2002). Profile, spectrum and significance of HBV genotypes in chronic liver disease patients in the Indian subcontinent. J Gastroenterol Hepatol. 17(2): 165-70.

[57] Tran et al. (2008) New complex recombinant genotype of hepatitis B virus identified in Vietnam. J Virol. 82(11):5657-63.

[58] Olinger C et al. (2008) Possible new hepatitis B virus genotype, Southeast Asia. Emerg Infect Dis. 14(11):1777-80.

[59] Tatematsu et al. (2009) A genetic variant of hepatitis B virus divergent from known human and ape genotypes isolated from a Japanese patient and provisionally assigned to new genotype J. J Virol. 83(20):10538-47.

[60] Mizokami M et al. (1999) Hepatitis B virus genotype assignment using restriction fragment length polymorphism patterns. FEBS Lett. 450(1-2):66-71.

[61] Farazmandfar T et al. (2012) A rapid and reliable genotyping method for hepatitis B virus genotypes (A-H) using type-specific primers. J Virol Methods. 181(1):114-6.

[62] Liu et al. (2008) Genotyping of hepatitis B virus genotypes A to G by multiplex polymerase chain reaction. Intervirology. 51(4):247-52.

[63] Chen J et al. (2007). Improved multiplex-PCR to identify hepatitis B virus genotypes A-F and subgenotypes B1, B2, C1 and C2. J Clin Virol. 38(3):238-43.

[64] Teles SA et al. (1999) Hepatitis B Virus: genotypes and subtypes in Brazilian hemodialysis patients. Artif Organs. 23(12):1074-8.

[65] Welzel TM et al. (2006) Real-time PCR assay for detection and quantification of hepatitis B virus genotypes A to G. J Clin Microbiol. 44(9):3325-33.

[66] Ganova-Raeva L et al. (2010) Robust hepatitis B virus genotyping by mass spectrometry. J Clin Microbiol. 48(11):4161-8.

[67] Guirgis BS et al. (2010) Hepatitis B virus genotyping: current methods and clinical implications. Int J Infect Dis. 14(11):941-53.

[68] Bartholomeusz A and Schaefer S (2004) Hepatitis B virus genotypes: comparison of genotyping methods. Rev Med Virol. 14(1):3-16.

[69] Echevarria JM and Avellon A (2006) Hepatitis B Virus genetic diversity. J Med Virol. 78(1):36-42.

[70] Schaefer S (2005) Hepatitis B virus: significance of genotypes. J Viral Hepat. 12(2):111-24.

[71] Janssen HL et al. (2005) Pegylated interferon alfa-2b alone or in combination with lamivudine for HBeAg-positive chronic hepatitis B: a randomized trial. Lancet. 65(9454):123- 9.

[72] Kao JH et al. (2002) Genotypes and clinical phenotypes of hepatitis B virus in patients with chronic hepatitis B virus infection. J Clin Microbiol. 40(4):1207- 9.

[73] Livingston SE et al (2007). Clearance of hepatitis B e antigen in patients with chronic hepatitis B and genotypes A, B, C, D, and F. Gastroenterology. 133(5):1452-7.

[74] Whalley SA et al. (2001). Kinetics of acute hepatitis B virus infection in humans. J Exp Med. 193(7):847-54.

[75] Girones R and Miller RH (1989) Mutation rate of the hepadnavirus genome. Virology. 170(2):595-7.

[76] Nowak MA et al. (1996) Viral dynamics in hepatitis B virus infections. Proc Natl Acad Sci U S A. 93(9):4398-402.

[77] Park SG et al. (2003) Fidelity of hepatitis B virus polymerase. Eur J Biochem. 270(14):2929-36.

[78] Locarnini S et al. (2003) The hepatitis B virus and common mutants. Semin Liver Dis. 23(1):5-20.

[79] Mizpkami M et al. (1997) Constrained evolution with respect to gene overlap of hepatitis B virus. J Mol Evol. 44 (1):S83-90.

[80] McMahon BJ (2010) Natural history of chronic hepatitis B. Clin Liver Dis 14(3):381-96.

[81] Wieland SF et al. (2005) Interferon prevents formation of replication-competent hepatitis B virus RNA-containing nucleocapsids. Proc Natl Acad Sci USA. 102(28):9913-17.

[82] Perrillo RP (2005) Current treatment of chronic hepatitis B: benefits and limitations. Semin. Liver Dis. 25(1):20-28.

[83] Zoulim F (2004) Antiviral therapy of chronic hepatitis B: can we clear the virus and prevent drug resistance? Antivir Chem Chemother. 15(6):299-305.

[84] Sung JJ et al. (2005) Intrahepatic hepatitis B virus covalently closed circular DNA can be a predictor of sustained response to therapy. Gastroenterology . 128(7):1890-97.

Chapter 4

An Overview of the Immune Evasion Strategies Adopted by Different Viruses with Special Reference to Classical Swine Fever Virus

S. Chakraborty, B.M. Veeregowda, R. Deb, and B.M. Chandra Naik

Additional information is available at the end of the chapter

http://dx.doi.org/10.5772/55435

1. Introduction

Viruses are considered as extremely successful predators as they can replicate and control the host cell synthesizing machinery. Viruses have coevolved with their hosts and thus have limited pathogenicity in any immunocompromised natural host. Viruses can exist in two forms: extra cellular virion particles and intracellular genomes. Virions are more resistant to physical stress than genomes but are susceptible to humoral immune control. Nevertheless, to exist as a species, virus replication and transfer to a new host are essential. These processes are associated with the production of antigenic proteins that make the virus vulnerable to immune control mechanisms 'warning' the host of the presence of an invader [1]. There are two classes of viral immunoregulatory proteins: the proteins encoded by genes having sequence similarity with cellular genes and those coded by genes without any sequence similarity to cellular genes. The second class of protein may represent a paradigm for co-evolution [2]. During the period of coexistence with their hosts, viruses have learned how to manipulate host immune control mechanism. It is well established that the viruses have evolved wide variety of immune evasion strategies *viz.,* evasion by noncytocidal infection (Arena and Hanta viruses), evasion by cell to cell spread (Canine distemper virus and cytomegalovirus), evasion by infection of nonpermissive, resting or undifferentiated cells (herpes virus induced latency), evasion by infection with restricted viral gene expression by destruction of immune effector cells and macrophages (destruction of $CD4^{+}$ T lymphocytes by HIV 1 and 2 viruses), evasion by downregulation of MHC – antigen expression (betaherpesviruses), evasion from cytokine action (Adenoviral infected cells evade the action of TNF through viral gene products), masking of epitopes and immune decoy (Ebola virus), evasion by induction of nonneutralizing antibodies (Aleutian Mink disease virus), evasion by induction of immunologic tolerance (congenital infections like Bovine Viral diarrhea, arena virus infections and some retro virus infections), evasion by sequestration in immunologically privileged tissues (replication of cytomegaloviruses in the kidney, salivary glands and mammary glands), evasion by integration of viral genome into host cell genome (induction of prophage in case of retro viral infection) and evasion by genetic drift (Maedi/Visna, Equine Infectious Anaemia) [2, 3]. The present review will highlight the different complex mechanisms associated with the host immune evasion by the viruses with special reference to the Classical Swine Fever Virus.

2. Newer concepts in the evasion of host deffense by viruses

The main sensors of the innate immune response are pattern recognition receptors (PRR) which can recognize pathogen associated molecular patterns (PAMPs). This recognition leads to the expression of cytokines, chemokines and co-stimulatory molecules that eliminate pathogens like viruses for the activation of antigen presenting cells and for the activation of specific adaptive response [4]. Among the PRRs, there are Toll Like Receptors (TLRs) that can be either endosomal or extracellular [5, 6] and retinoic acid-inducible gene-(RIG-)I/MDA5 (melanoma differentiation-associated gene) [7] known as RNA helicase-like receptors (RLRs). Further, Double-stranded RNA-dependent protein kinase (PKR), 2', 5'-oligoadenylate synthetase (2'- 5' OAS), and adenosine deaminase acting on RNA (ADAR), known as effector proteins, complement the function of PRRs. All these proteins are responsible for recognizing viral components and induce proinflammatory cytokine expression or interferon (IFN) response factors. There are certain cellular components which are manipulated by viruses to evade the innate immune response. Expression of type-I IFN depends on the activation of Interferon Regulatory Factor - 3 (IRF3) and IRF7 via I kappa B kinase (IKK) epsilon and Tank Binding Kinase 1 (TBK1). The genome of Rabies virus, Borna disease virus and Ebola virus code for the P phosphoprotein and VP35 that can block the antiviral response induced by IFN [8, 9, 10]. In contrast, the human herpes simplex virus 8 encodes different analogs of IRF with negative dominant activity, allowing it to interfere with the activity of cellular IRFs [11]. The infected cell polypeptide 0 (ICP0) from Bovine herpes virus can interact with IRF3 and induce its proteasome-dependent degradation [12]. Similarly, the V protein of paramyxoviruses interacts with MD5-α and inhibits IFN-α expression [13].

One of the major non-speific humoral deffense mechanisms of the body for combating and clearing the infectious agents is complement system [14, 15, 16]. Viruses encode homologs of complement regulatory proteins that are secreted and block complement activation and neutralization of virus particles. The cowpox virus (CPV) complement inhibitor, termed inflammation modulatory protein (IMP), blocks immunopathological tissue damage at the site of infection, presumably by inhibiting production of the macrophage chemo attractant factors C3a and C5a. Viruses protect the membranes of infected cells and the lipid envelopes of virus particles from complement lysis by encoding homologs of inhibitors of the membrane-attack complex. Human cytomegalovirus (HCMV), HIV and vaccinia virus (VV) used to borrow different host cellular factors, such as CD59, to protect from complement action. Moreover, some viruses encode Fc receptors [17], thus inducing antibody response.

These antibodies may kill infected cells by complement-mediated cytolysis or by antibody-dependent cell-mediated cytotoxicity (ADCC).

In case of FMD virus, following a 5' untranslated region known as the S fragment, there is poly "C" tract comprising over 90 per cent 'C' residues [18]. The length of this tract is extremely variable [19]. There are some evidences that length of this tract is associated with virulence and persistence of infections [20].

There is also evidence of viral interference with interferons. Interferons were discovered because of their ability to protect cells from viral infection. The key role of both type I (α and β) and type II (γ) IFNs as one of the first anti-viral defense mechanisms is indicated by the fact that anti-IFN strategies are present in most viruses. Viruses block IFN-induced transcriptional responses and the Janus Kinase (JAK) / signal transducers and activators of transcription (STAT) signal transduction pathways also inhibit the activation of IFN effector pathways that induce an anti-viral state in the cell and limit virus replication. This is mainly achieved by inhibiting double-stranded (ds)-RNA-dependent protein kinase (PKR) activation. Once active, the PKR causes phosphorylation of eukaryotic translation initiation factor 2a (eIF-2a) and the RNase L system, which are responsible for degrading viral RNA and translation in the host cell. Moreover, active PKR is also able to mediate the activation of the transcription factor NFkB which upregulates the expression of interferon cytokines, which work to spread the antiviral signal locally. In addition, active PKR is also able to induce cellular apoptosis. All these mechanisms due to PKR activation ultimately leads to inhibition of the spread of viral infection. But inhibition of PKR activation causes the viral infection to spread and thus helps in evasion of the immune system. Secreted cytokine receptors or binding proteins are mainly encoded by Poxviruses which actually encode soluble versions of receptors for IFN-α and -β (IFN-α/bR) and IFN-γ (IFN-γR), which also block the immune functions of IFNs 6. The IFN-α/βR secreted by Vaccinia virus (VV) is also localized at the cell surface to protect cells from IFN [21, 22]. Additionally, several viruses inhibit the activity of IFN-γ, a key activator of cellular immunity, by blocking the synthesis or activity of factors required for its production, such as interleukin (IL)-18 or IL-12. CPV cytokine response modifier (Crm) A inhibits caspase-1, which processes the mature forms of IL-1b and IL-18 [23]; various poxviruses encode soluble IL-18-binding proteins (IL-18BPs) [24]; measles virus (MeV) binds CD46 in macrophages and inhibits IL-12 production [15]; herpes viruses and poxviruses express IL-10 homologs that diminish the Th1 response by downregulating the production of IL-12 [25, 26].

Cytokines play a key role in the initiation and regulation of the innate and adaptive immune responses, and viruses have learned how to block cytokine production, activity and signal transduction. African swine fever virus (ASFV) replicates in macrophages and encodes an IkB homolog that blocks cytokine expression mediated by nuclear factor (NF)-kB and the nuclear factor activated T cell (NFAT) transcription factors 13. Many viruses block signal transduction by ligands of the tumor necrosis factor (TNF) family, whereas others deliberately induce some cytokine pathways; For example, the Epstein–Barr virus (EBV) latent membrane protein 1 (LMP1) recruits components of the TNF receptor (TNFR) and CD40 transduction machinery to mimic cytokine responses that could be beneficial for the virus, such as cell proliferation [27]. One of the most interesting mechanisms identified in recent years is the mimicry of cytokines (virokines) and cytokine receptors (viroceptors) by large DNA viruses like herpesviruses and poxviruses [28, 29]. The functions of these molecules in the animal host are diverse. Soluble viral cytokine receptors might neutralize cytokine activity and cytokine homologs might redirect the immune response for the benefit of the virus. Alternatively, viruses that infect immune cells might use these homologs to induce signalling pathways in the infected cell that promote virus replication. The herpesvirus cytokine homologs vIL-6 and vIL-17 might have immunomodulatory activity but might also increase proliferation of cells that are targets for viral replication [28]. Viral semaphoring homologs have uncovered a role for the semaphorin family, previously known as chemoattractants or chemorepellents involved in axonal guidance during development in the immune system, and have identified a semaphorin receptor in macrophages that mediates cytokine production [30, 31].

Apoptosis, or programmed cell death, can be triggered by a variety of inducers, including ligands of the TNF family, irradiation, cell cycle inhibitors or infectious agents such as viruses. The cellular proteins implicated in the control of apoptosis are targeted by viral anti-apoptotic mechanisms [32, 33]. Viruses inhibit activation of caspases: encode homologs of the anti-apoptotic protein Bcl-2, block apoptotic signals triggered by activation of TNFR family members by encoding death-effector-domain-containing proteins and inactivate IFN-induced PKR and the tumor suppressor p53, both of which promote apoptosis. Epstein-Barr virus and oncogenic human herpes viruses use Bcl-2 orthologs like BHRF1 and BALF-1 to block mitochondrial release of cytochrome c [34, 35]. Mouse γ- herpesvirus (MHV) -68 encodes a Bcl-2 ortholog (MHVBcl-2) that protects the infected cell against TNF-mediated apoptosis [36]. An alternative mechanism is provided by the glutathione peroxidase of molluscum contagiosum virus (MCV), which provides protection from peroxide or UV induced apoptosis and perhaps from peroxides induced by TNF, macrophages or neutrophils.

Infection with the human and simian immunodeficiency viruses are unique in that the infections give rise to prolonged, continuous viral replication in the infected host. Destruction of virus-specific T helper cells, the emergence of antigenic escape variants and the expression of an envelope complex that structurally minimizes antibody escape to conserved epitopes contribute to persistence. Moreover, the virus encoded protein Nef prevents the viral antigen presentation [37].

3. Recognition of CSFV by immune system

Amidst the diversified mechanisms evolved by different viruses to evade the host immunity (innate or adaptive), CSFV plays a unique role in evading the host deffense and maintain the infection. The virus expresses two major PAMPs: the ssRNA genome and the dsRNA replication intermediates. The TLR's sensing such patterns are located in the endosomal compartment [38] or in the cytoplasm in case of the cellular helicases Retinoic acid-Inducible Gene 1 (RIG-I) and Melanoma Differentiation-Associated protein 5 (MDA-5) [39]. TLR3 binds dsRNA [40, 41], whereas TLR7 recognizes ssRNA [42, 43]. Conventional DC mainly expresses TLR3 [44] while plasmacytoid DC (pDC) express TLR7 [45]. RIG-I and MDA-5 both bind dsRNA. Recently however it was shown that RIG-I can sense uncapped viral single stranded RNA bearing a 5'-triphosphate [46, 47]. The stimulation of TLR3 leads to the activation of NFkB (early NFkB response) or to the activation of IRF3, which in turn upregulates type I IFN transcription and subsequently transcription of NFkB (late NFkB response) [48]. TLR7 stimulation leads to the activation of IRF7 but not of IRF3 [49]. Thus there is induction of type I interferons and various pro-inflammatory cytokines which play crucial role in antiviral host immune responses. Understimulation of any of these two TLR's (*i,e.,* either TLR 3 or 7) leads to down regulation of host immune response and over stimulation leads to exaggerated immune response.

4. Few salient features about the disease Classical Swine Fever

Classical swine fever (CSF) is a disease of domestic pigs and wild boar caused by CSF virus (CSFV). CSFV, first reported in the United States in 1833 causes important economical losses worldwide. Besides the United States of America, only Australia, Canada, Ireland, New Zealand, the Scandinavian countries and Switzerland are currently considered free of CSFV. In Europe the recent outbreaks occurred in Bulgaria Croatia and Germany in the year 2006 [50].

The natural reservoir for CSFV is the wild boar, which remains the major threat for new outbreaks. The virus is endemic in most of the Eastern European countries but the domestic pig population of Western Europe can be considered free from the disease. The control measures for CSFV include stamping out with a non-vaccination policy. Consequently pigs have to be free of virus and antibody against CSFV. Whether seroconversion results from vaccination or disease, pigs seropositive for CSFV must be eliminated. Acute or endemic CSF in domestic pigs has large economic impact on general restriction on pig meat trade [51]. The outbreak of CSF, and occurrences of CSFV in the tissues of pigs were reported from India as well [52].

There are three distinct genogroups of the virus (*viz.,* 1, 2 and 3) with three or four subgroups [53, 54]. Even though group 1 viruses are predominant in India, group 2 viruses are also rapidly spreading and may form a major threat in future [55].

Early stage of the disease (CSF) is characterized by fever and diarrhoea. The gradual progression of the disease results in a severe wasting syndrome. The terminal stage is signified by a blue discoloration of the skin and weakness of the hind legs along with neurological symptoms. Autopsy finding includes disseminated intravascular coagulopathy, extensive tissue hemorrhages and thymus atrophy [56].

5. A few salient features of the structure, composition and function of the CSFV genome

Classical swine fever virus (CSFV) is a member of the family *Flaviviridae,* genus *Pestivirus* [57]. The species consist of small, spherical enveloped viruses with an approximate diameter of 40-60 nm based around an electron-dense inner core structure of about 30 nm [58]. The virus bears a single stranded positive sense RNA molecule spanning approximately 12.5 kbp and is made up of a single open reading frame (ORF) flanked by a 3' and 5' nontranslated region (NTR), the latter contains conserved regions implicated in the translational events [59, 60]. Notwithstanding the fact that the virus has a RNA genome, it is reported to be relatively stable [61]. Nevertheless, a recent study [62] indicated that recombination between strains is possible. The ORF is translated into a single polypeptide of about 3900 amino acids which is co-and post-translationally processed into mature peptide by a number of virus and host encoded proteases [63, 64, 65, 66]. The virion is made up of 4 structural proteins *viz.*, C, Erns, E1 and E2 which are encoded at the 5' end of the genome. The spherical nucleocapsid coat of the virus is composed of numerous proteins while the surface is made out of Erns, E1 and E2 in homodimeric (Erns, E2) or heterodimeric (E1E2) form [67, 68]. E1 and E2 consist of transmembrane domains whereas Erns has no transmembrane spanning domain and its attachment to the virion is rather tenuous. In addition to the structural proteins, the CSFV viral genome encodes further 8 non-structural proteins, including an N-terminal protease (Npro), p7, the non-structural proteins (NS) 2, 3, 4A, 4B, 5A and finally 5B [64, 69].

CSFV is normally a noncytopathogenic (ncp) virus. A rare cytopathogenic (cp) form can occur spontaneously in cell culture [70] and has also been found in wild boar [71]. Its significance in CSFV pathogenesis is unknown. The CSFV genome consists of single stranded positive sense RNA. This RNA carries a single large open reading frame (ORF) flanked by a 5' and a 3' non-translated region (NTR). The NTR at the 5' end harbours an internal ribosome entry site [72, 73, 74]. Therefore the RNA can directly undergo cap independent translation upon uncoating. The large ORF encodes a single polyprotein which is co and post-translationally cleaved into altogether 12 structural and non-structural proteins including N^{pro} (the first protein encoded by the ORF) by either cellular signalases or viral proteases [75]. It exhibits auto protease activity and cleaves itself from the nascent polyprotein [76]. N^{pro} is the only viral gene that can be deleted without altering virus replication [77]. There is also report of counteraction of the type I IFN induction pathway by N^{pro} [78, 79, 80] by down-regulating the expression levels of the interferon regulatory factor 3 (IRF3) [81, 82]. IRF3 is the rate limiting component of the INF-b promotor enhanceosome and thus regulates the transcriptional activity of this gene [83, 84]. The second protein translated by the ORF is the capsid protein C (Core). It contains the E^{rns} signal sequence [85] and a signalase recognition site [86]. The C gene is followed by the other three structural genes Erns, E1 and E2, the three envelope proteins of CSFV. All these proteins are cleaved by signalases [86]. E^{rns} exists in secreted form [87]. It exhibits RNase activity *in vitro* [85]. It remains unclear whether this RNase activity has a specific role in the life cycle of CSFV. A lymphotoxic function of the secreted Erns has been reported [88]. More recently it has been shown that Erns of BVDV is involved in the inhibition of dsRNA-mediated type I IFN induction [89]. A very recent report proposed a cooperative effect of N^{pro} and Erns of BVDV on transplacental infection in cattle [90]. Encoded downstream of envelope protein gene E1, the glycoprotein E2 harbours the major immunogenic epitopes. The antigenic region of E2 was divided in the three domains A, B and C based on analysis using monoclonal antibodies (mAb) [91, 92]. E1 and E2 form either homodimers or heterodimers. They both contain transmembrane regions that anchor the glycoproteins in the viral envelope. Erns has no transmembrane region and is associated with the envelope by interaction with E1 and/or E2 or by hydrophobic interactions with the membrane. The p7 protein is not part of the virion but was found to be essential for virus assembly [93]. Protein p7 of the closely related hepatitis C virus (HCV) forms an ion channel [94]. It is not clear yet whether p7 of CSFV has the same function. The non-structural gene products are cleaved by the NS2 autoprotease between NS2 and NS3 [95] and by the NS3 protease at the downstream cleavage sites [96, 97, 98]. NS2 is an inducible autoprotease that is activated by four cellular proteins [99, 100]. Enhanced cleavage between NS2 and NS3 correlates with the appearance of the cp biotype [101]. The uncleaved NS2-3 protein is essential for the formation of viral particles [101, 102]. The cleaved NS3 protein is produced essentially during the first few hours post-infection. Besides being a protease the NS3 protein has also helicase [103, 104] and NTPase activity [105, 106]. The NS4A protein is an essential co-factor of the NS3 protease [107]. NS4B is assumed to be a co-factor of the RNA-dependent RNA-polymerase encoded by the NS5B gene. This RNA-polymerase contains a GDD (Glycine-D-aspartate-D-aspartate) active site motif, otherwise known as the motif c [108]. The binding and entry of pestiviruses is a multistep process involving initial attachment of virions, interaction with specific receptor(s), internalization, and membrane fusion [109, 110, 111, 112]. The surface protein CD46 was proposed as receptor for BVDV [104]. Specific cell surface receptors for CSFV have not yet been identified. It has been shown that recombinant E2, E1 and Erns can independently bind to the cell surface [113, 114]. E2 adsorption competitively inhibits infection with homotypic and heterotypic pestiviruses [115]. After capsid uncoating, RNA replication and translation takes place in so-called replication complexes. These complexes have been well characterized for the closely related hepatitis C virus [116] and for some members of the genus Flavivirus [117]. The assembly pathway of pestiviruses is poorly understood. As mentioned above the uncleaved NS2-3 precursor protein in association with NS4A are essential for particles formation [101, 118]. Several studies on different pestiviruses have revealed that NS4B is an endoplasmic reticulum (ER)-associated integral membrane protein that contains four putative transmembrane domains flanked by cytoplasmic N- and C-terminal regions [119, 120, 121, 122]. Interaction of CSFV NS4B with molecular components of the immune system has also been reported [123].

6. N^{pro} and its role in induction of poly (IC) induced antiviral activities

The first protein encoded is the non-structural protein N^{pro}. The gene coding for this protein is the only non-essential gene in the pestivirus life cycle [124]. It exhibits autoproteolytical activity and cleaves itself off the downstream nucleocapsid protein C [125, 126, 127]. When CSFV, BVDV and BDV are compared, the amino acid sequence identity of N^{pro} is found to be higher than 70 per cent [128] and the residues Glu22, His49, and Cys69 are essential for the proteiolytic activity of N^{pro} [125]. Moreover, the residues Cys168 and Ser 169 surrounding the cleavage sites are also conserved [126]. Resistance to poly(IC)-induced cell death and control of IFN induction are dependent on the presence of the N^{pro} gene, indicating a function of N^{pro} in innate immune evasion of CSFV [129]. The characterisation of N^{pro} gene is also found to be beneficial for the development of inactivated vaccine [130].

7. Immune evasion and immunopathogenesis of CSF

CSF virus (CSFV) has high affinity for vascular endothelial cells and lymphoreticular cells including T cells, B cells and monocytes [122]. Severe depletion of B cells and T cells in Peripheral Blood Mononuclear Cells (PBMC) and virus persistence in lymphoid tissues is thought to be the most important characteristics of CSFV infection that leads to the acquired immunosuppressive state [131, 132].

Recently it has been observed that ncp BVDV induces translocation of IRF-3 into the nucleus without subsequent binding to DNA [133]. Furthermore, ncp BVDV was able to block Semliki Forest virus-induced IFN production through a block in the formation of IRF-3 – DNA complexes [134]. Whether this is also true for CSFV and whether N^{pro} is involved in this process remain to be investigated. But we can not ignore the fact that the presence of N^{pro} permits efficient infection of monocytic cells, including monocytes, macrophages, and even dendritic cells.These cells are among the main targets for CSFV allowing high-level replication and permit cell-associated spreading and colonization of immunological tissue by CSFV. Furthermore, they appear to play a central role in virus-induced immunomodulation [135].

Dendritic cells (DCs) are one of the primary immunological sentinels of the immune system [136, 137]. Their strategic localization at mucosal surfaces and dermal layers makes them an early target for virus contact [138]. Functional disruption of DCs is an important strategy for viral pathogens to evade host defences [139, 140]. Monocytotropic viruses such as CSFV can employ such a mechanism as the virus can suppress immune responses and induce apoptosis without infecting lymphocytes. The virus infects both conventional dendritic cells (cDCs) and plasmacytoid dendritic cells (pDCs) [141, 142, 143]. The infected DCs display neither modulated MHC nor CD80/86 expression. Interestingly, similar to macrophages, CSFV do not induce IFN-α responses in the cDCs as N^{pro} protein promotes proteosomal degradation of interferon regulatory factor (IRF) 3 [144, 145]. So, it can be said that CSFV can replicate in cDCs and control type I IFN responses, without interfering with the immune reactivity [146]. However, in pDCs, IRF 7 is more prominent and there is lack of interference of N^{pro} with IRF 3 which results in augmented IFN α response by pDCs. This is the reason for an exaggerated pDC response, relating to the immunopathological characteristics of the disease [147, 148, 149].

Regulation of CSFV RNA turnover with minimal accumulation of dsRNA is an important factor governing the evasion of host deffense by the virus [144]. The temporal modulation of NS2-3 processing by the NS2 autoprotease is crucial in RNA replication control and the intracellular level of NS3 strictly correlates with the efficiency of RNA replication [150]. But, whether these proteins regulate the dsRNA levels remains to be established. The viral structural protein E^{rns} is also actively involved in the dsRNA-mediated induction of IFNβ [151].

IL-6 is an important cytokine in providing protection during early part of CSFV infection. The synthesis of NS4B protein during viral replication in the tonsil down regulates the expression of IL-6 and this is especially true with CSFV strain Brescia [123]. Swine

Leukocyte Antigen I (SLA I) molecules present the endogenous peptides to activate the $CD8^+$ T cells that control viral replication within cells. CSFV interferes with the expression of SLA I molecules by the monocytic cells, thereby, inhibiting apoptosis of the cells. This strategy seems to be quiet helpful for the virus to escape the host immuno-surveillance and establishment of persistence in tissues [152]. Antibodies may be temporarily detected in serum sample. But these antibodies can not eliminate the virus from the host system. Consequently, the antibodies are neutralized by the virus and cease to be detectable [153].

Blocking B-lymphocyte maturation by infection and destruction of germinal centers is a key event in the pathogenesis of acute, lethal CSF before the development of generalized infection [154]. Immature B lymphocytes (*i,e.,* centroblasts, centrocytes and B blasts) can themselves be the cellular targets of the virus in any stage of maturation within follicles [155] or they may lack critical cytokines because of an infection of the supporting follicular dendritic cell network [154]. However, it is clear that depletion of B lymphocytes can not account for all the pleiotropic symptoms of this disease. But, as it is generally held that antibodies against CSF can be protective and as recovery from acute infection is known to be associated with seroconversion [156, 157] it appears justified that B-follicle tropism of an HCV isolate is an important determinant for the course of disease [154].

8. Conclusion

The understanding of the virus-host interaction network is important to design antiviral strategies and to formulate antiviral drugs. In this context, the ability of the viruses to evade the host immune system plays a key role. The understanding of the complex mechanisms of host immune system manipulation will ultimately result in undertaking suitable immunoprohylactic measures.

Author details

S. Chakraborty
M.V.Sc (Veterinary Microbiology), Veterinary College, Hebbal, Bengaluru, Karnataka, India

B. M. Veeregowda
Dept. of Veterinary Microbiology, Veterinary College, Hebbal, Bengaluru, Karnataka

R. Deb
Project Directorate on Cattle, Meerut, U. P, India

B. M. Chandra Naik
Dept. of Veterinary Microbiology, Veterinary College, Hebbal, Bengaluru, Karnataka, India

9. References

[1] Pulendran, B., Palucka, K. & Banchereau, J. (2001). Sensing pathogens and tuning immune responses. *Sci.,* 293: 253–256.

[2] MacLachlan, N. J. and Dubovi, E. J. Fenner's Veterinary Virology. 4th Edition.
[3] White, D. O. and Fenner, F. J. Medical Virology. 4th Edition.
[4] Pedraza, S. T., Betancur, J. G. and Urcuqui-Inchima, S. (2010). Viral recognition by the innate immune system: the role of pattern recognition receptors. *Colomb. Med.,* 41(4): 377-387.
[5] Janeway C. and Medzhitov R. (2000). Viral interference with IL-1 and toll signalling. *Proc. Natl. Acad. Sci.,* 97: 10682-10683.
[6] Netea, M. G., van der Graaf, C., Van der Meer, J. W. and Kullberg, B. J. (2004). Toll-like receptors and the host defense against microbial pathogens: bringing specificity to the innate-immune system. *J. Leukoc. Biol.,* 75: 749-755.
[7] Kang, J. Y, Nan, X., Jin, M. S, Youn, S. J., Ryu, Y. H. and Mah, S. (2009). Recognition of lipopeptide patterns by Toll-like receptor 2- Toll-like receptor 6 heterodimer. *Immunity.* 31: 873-884.
[8] Brzozka, K., Finke, S. and Conzelmann K. K. (2005). Identification of the rabies virus alpha/beta interferon antagonist: phosphoprotein P interferes with phosphorylation of interferon regulatory factor 3. *J. Virol.,* 79: 7673-7681.
[9] Conzelmann, K. K. (2005). Transcriptional activation of alpha/beta interferon genes: interference by non-segmented negative strand RNA viruses. *J. Virol.,* 79: 5241-5248.
[10] Feng, Z., Cerveny, M., Yan, Z. and He, B. (2007). The VP35 protein of Ebola virus inhibits the antiviral effect mediated by double-stranded RNA-dependent protein kinase PKR. *J. Virol.,* 81: 182-192.
[11] Lin, R., Genin, P., Mamane, Y., Sgarbanti, M., Battistini, A. and Harrington, W. J. (2001). HHV-8 encoded vIRF-1 represses the interferon antiviral response by blocking IRF-3 recruitment of the CBP/p300 co activators. *Oncogene.* 20: 800-11.
[12] Saira K., Zhou Y. and Jones C. (2007). The infected cell protein 0 encoded by bovine herpesvirus 1 (bICP0) induces degradation of interferon response factor 3 and, consequently, inhibits beta interferon promoter activity. *J. Virol.,* 81: 3077-3086.
[13] Andrejeva, J., Childs, K. S., Young, D. F., Carlos, T. S., Stock, N. and Goodbourn, S. (2004). The V proteins of paramyxoviruses bind the IFN-inducible RNA helicase, mda-5, and inhibit its activation of the IFN-beta promoter. *Proc. Natl. Acad. Sci.,* 101: 17264-17269.
[14] Smith, G. L., Symons, J. A., Khanna, A., Vanderplasschen, A. and Alcami, A. (1997). Vaccinia virus immune evasion. *Immunol. Rev.,* 159: 137–154.
[15] Tortorella, D., Benjamin, E. G., Margo, H. F., Danny, J. S. and Hidde, L. P. (2000). Viral subversion of the immune system. *Annu. Rev. Immunol.,* 18: 861–926.
[16] Kotwal, G. J. (2000). Poxviral mimicry of complement and chemokine system components: what's the end game? *Immunol. Today* 21: 242–248.
[17] Kalvakolanu, D.V. (1999). Virus interception of cytokine-regulated pathways. *Trends Microbiol.,* 7: 166–171.
[18] Longjam, N., Deb, R., Sarmah, A. K., Tayo, T., Awachat, V. B. and Saxena, V. K. (2011). A brief review on diagnosis of Foot-and-Mouth disease of livestock: Conventional to molecular tools. *Vet. Med. Int.,* 1-17.

[19] Giomi, M. P. C., Bergmann, I. E. and Scodeller, E. A. (1984). Heterogeneity of the polyribocytidylic acid tract in aphthovirus: biochemical and biological studies of viruses carrying polyribocytidylic acid tracts of different lengths. *J. Virol.*, 51: 799–805.

[20] Harris, T. J. R. and Brown, F. (1977). Biochemical analysis of a virulent and an avirulent strain of foot and mouth disease virus. *J. Gen. Virol.*, 34(1): 87–105.

[21] Smith, G. L., Symons, J. A. and Alcami, A. (1998). Poxviruses: interfering with interferons. *Sem. Virol.*, 8: 409–418.

[22] Goodbourn, S., Didcock, L. and Randall, R. E. (2000). Interferons: cell signalling, immune modulation, antiviral responses and virus countermeasures. *J. Gen. Virol., 81: 2341-2364.*

[23] Xiang, Y. and Moss, B. (1999). IL-18 binding and inhibition of interferon gamma induction by human poxvirus-encoded proteins. *Proc. Natl. Acad. Sci.*, 96: 11537–11542.

[24] Born, T. L., Morrison, L. A., Esteban, D. J., Vandenbos, T., Thebeau, L. G., Chen, N., Spriggs, M. K., Sims, J. E. and Buller, R. M. L. (2000). A poxvirus protein that binds to and inactivates IL-18 and inhibits NK cell response. *J. Immunol.*, 164: 3246–3254.

[25] Spriggs, M. K. (1996). One step ahead of the game: viral immunomodulatory molecules. *Annu. Rev. Immunol.*, 14: 101–130.

[26] Kotenko, S. V., Saccani, S., Izotova, L. S., Mirochnitchenko, O. V. and Pestka, S. (2000). Human cytomegalovirus harbors its own unique IL-10 homolog (cmvIL-10). *Proc. Natl. Acad. Sci., U. S. A.* 97: 1695–1700.

[27] Farrell, P. J. (1998). Signal transduction from the Epstein–Barr virus LMP-1 transforming protein. *Trends. Microbiol.*, 6: 175–177.

[28] Nash, P., Barrett, J. and Cao, J. X. (1999). Immunomodulation by viruses: the myxoma virus story. *Immunol. Rev.*, 168: 103–120.

[29] Lalani, A. S., Barrett, J. W. and McFadden, G. (2000). Modulating chemokines: more lessons from viruses. *Immunol. Today* 21: 100–106.

[30] Spriggs, M. K. (1999). Shared resources between the neural and immune systems: semaphorins join the ranks. *Curr. Opin. Immunol.*, 11: 387–391.

[31] Alcami, A. and Koszinowski, U.H. (1998). Poxviruses: capturing cytokines and chemokines. *Sem. Virol.*, 8: 419–427.

[32] Turner, P. C. and Moyer, R. W. (1998). Control of apoptosis by poxviruses. *Sem. Virol.*, 8: 453–469.

[33] Everett, H. and McFadden, G. (1999). Apoptosis: an innate immune response to virus infection. *Trends Microbiol.*, 7: 160–165.

[34] Henderson, S. (1993). Epstein-Barr virus-coded BHRF I protein, a viral homologue of Bcl-2, protect human B cells from programmed cell death. *Proc. Natl. Acad. Sci.*, 90: 8479-8483.

[35] Marshall, W. L., Datta, R., Hanify, K., Teng, E. and Finberg, R. W. (1999). U937 cells over expressing bcl-xl are resistant to human immunodefficiency virus-I induced apoptosis and human immunodeficiency virus-I replication. *Virol.*, 256: 1-7.

[36] Benedict, C. A., Norris, P. S. and Ware, C. F. (2002). To kill or be killed: viral evasion of apoptosis. Nature. 3(11): 1013-1018.

[37] Johnson, W. E. and Desrosiers, R. C. (2002). Viral Persistence: HIV's strategies of immune system evasion. *Annu. Rev. Med.,* 53: 499 – 518.

[38] Kawai, T. and Akira, S. (2006). TLR signalling. *Cell Death. Differ.,* 13: 816-825.

[39] Yoneyama, M., Kikuchi, M., Matsumoto, K., Imaizumi, T., Miyagishi, M., Taira, K., Foy, E., Loo, Y.M., Gale, M., Akira, S., Yonehara, S., Kato, A. and Fujita, T. (2005). Shared and Unique Functions of the DExD/H-Box Helicases RIG-I, MDA5, and LGP2 in Antiviral Innate Immunity. *J. Immunol.,* 175: 2851-2858.

[40] Matsumoto, M., Funami, K., Oshiumi, H. and Seya, T. (2004). Toll-like receptor 3: A link between toll-like receptor, interferon and viruses. *Microbiol. Immunol.,* 48: 147-154.

[41] Sen, G.C. and Sarkar, S.N. (2005). Transcriptional signaling by double-stranded RNA: role of TLR3. *Cytokine Growth Factor Rev.,* 16: 1-14.

[42] Crozat, K. and Beutler, B. (2004). TLR7: A new sensor of viral infection. *Proc. Nat. Acad. Sci.,* 101: 6835-6836.

[43] Diebold, S. S., Kaisho, T., Hemmi, H., Akira, S. and Sousa, C. R. E. (2004). Innate antiviral responses by means of TLR7-mediated recognition of single-stranded RNA. *Scie.,* 303: 1529-1531.

[44] Visintin, A., Mazzoni, A., Spitzer, J. H., Wyllie, D. H., Dower, S. K. and Segal, D. M. (2001). Regulation of Toll-like receptors in human monocytes and dendritic cells. *J. Immunol.,* 166: 249-255.

[45] Ito, T., Wang, Y. H. and Liu, Y. J. (2005). Plasmacytoid dendritic cell precursors/type I interferon producing cells sense viral infection by Toll-like receptor (TLR) 7 and TLR9. *Springer Semin. Immunopathol.,* 26: 221-229.

[46] Hornung, V., Ellegast, J., Kim, S., Brzozka, K., Jung, A., Kato, H., Poeck, H., Akira, S., Conzelmann, K. K., Schlee, M., Endres, S. and Hartmann, G. (2006). 5'-Triphosphate RNA is the ligand for RIG-I. *Scie.,* 314: 994-997.

[47] Pichlmair, A., Schulz, O., Tan, C. P., Naslund, T. I., Liljestrom, P., Weber, F. and Reis, S. (2006). RIG-I-mediated antiviral responses to single-stranded RNA bearing 5'-phosphates. *Scie.,* 314: 997-1001.

[48] Akira, S. and Hemmi, H. (2003). Recognition of pathogen-associated molecular patterns by TLR family. *Immunol. Lett.,* 85: 85-95.

[49] Kawai, T., Sato, S., Ishii, K. J., Coban, C., Hemmi, H., Yamamoto, M., Terai, K., Matsuda, M., Inoue, J., Uematsu, S., Takeuchi, O. and Akira, S. (2004). Interferon-alpha induction through Toll-like receptors involves a direct interaction of IRF7 with MyD88 and TRAF6. *Nat. Immunol.,* 5: 1061-1068.

[50] Ruggli, N. and Summerfield, A. (2007). Characterization of immune evasion strategies of classical swine fever virus in monocytic and dendritic cells. Ph.D thesis, Institute of Virology and Immunoprophylaxis, Mittelhausern, Switzerland.

[51] http://www.oie.int/wahid.

[52] Sarma, D. K. and Bostami, B. (2008). Isolation and growth characteristics of classical swine fever in PK-15 cell line. *J. Appl. Biosci. Biotech.,* 3: 29–32.

[53] Lowings, P., Ibata, G., Needham, J. and Paton, D. (1996). Classical swine fever virus diversity and evolution. *J. Gen. Virol.,* 77: 1311-1321.

[54] Paton, D. J., McGoldrick, A., GreiserWilke, I., Parchariyanon, S., Song, J. Y., Liou, P. P., Stadejek, T., Lowings, J. P., Bjorklund, H. and Belak, S. (2000). Genetic typing of classical swine fever virus. *Vet. Microbiol.*, 73: 137-157.

[55] Chakraborty, S., Veeregowda, B. M., Chandra Naik, B. M., Rathnamma, D., Isloor, S., Venkatesha, M. D., Leena, G., Veeresh, H. and Patil, S. S. (2011). Molecular characterization and genogrouping of classical sine fever virus isolated from field outbreaks. *Ind. J. Anim. Sci.*, 81(8): 803-806.

[56] Trautwein, G. (1988). Pathology and pathogenesis of the disease, p. 27-53. In B. Liess (ed.), Classical swine fever and related viral infections. Martinus Nijhoff Publishing, Boston.

[57] Fauquet, C. M., Mayo, M. A., Maniloff, J., Desselberger, U. and Ball, L. A. (2005). Virus Taxonomy. Eighth Report of the International Committee on Taxonomy of Viruses. Academic Press, SanDiego.

[58] Moennig V., Floegel-Niesmann G. and Greiser-Wilke I. (2003). Clinical signs and epidemiology of classical swine fever: a review of new knowledge. *Vet J.*, 165(1): 11-20.

[59] Sizova, D. V., Kolupaeva, V. G., Pestova, T. V., Shatsky, I. N. and Hellen, C. U. T. (1998). Specific interaction eukaryotic translation initiation factor 3 with the 5' non translated regions of Hepatitis C virus and Classical Swine Fever Virus RNAs. *J. Virol.*, 72(6): 4775-4782.

[60] Fletcher, S. P. and Jackson, R. J. (2002). Pestivirus Internal Ribosome Entry Site (IRES) structure and function: Elements in the 5' untranslated region important for IRES function. *J. Virol.*, 76: 5024-5033.

[61] Vanderhallen, H., Mittelholzer, C., Hofmann, M. A. and Koenen, F. (1999). Classical swine fever virus is genetically stable in vitro and in vivo. *Arch. Virol.*, 144(9): 1669-1677.

[62] He, D. M., Qian, K. X., Shen, G. F., Zhang, Z. F., Li, Y. N., Su, Z. L. and Shao, H. B. (2007). Recombination and expression of classical swine fever virus (CSFV) structural protein E2 gene in *Chlamydomonas reinhardtii* chloroplasts. *Colloids and Surfaces B: Biointerfaces.*, 55(1): 26-30.

[63] Rümenapf, T., Unger, G., Strauss, J. H. and Thiel, H. J. (1993). Processing of the envelope glycoproteins of pestiviruses. *J. Virol.*, 67: 3288-3294.

[64] Falgout, B., Pethel, M. and Zhang, Y. M. (1995). Flaviviridae: The viruses and their replication. *J. Virol.*, 69(11): 7232-7243.

[65] Elbers, A. R. W., Stegeman, A., Moser, H., Ekker, H. M., Smak, J. A. and Pluimers, F. H. (1999). The classical swine fever epidemic197-1998 in the Netherlands: descriptive epidemiology. *Preventive Vet. Med.*, 42(3-4): 157-184.

[66] Heimann, M., Roman-Sosa, G., Martoglio, B., Thiel, H. J. and Rümenapf, T. (2006). Core protein of pestiviruses is processed at the C terminus by signal peptide peptidase. *J. Virol.*, 80: 1915-1921.

[67] Thiel, H. J., Stark, R., Meyers, G., Weiland, E. and Rumenapf, T. (1991). Proteins encoded in the 5′ region of the pestivirus genome – considerations concerning taxonomy. *Vet. Microbiol.*, 33: 213-219.

[68] König, M., Lengsfeld, T., Pauly, T., Stark, R. and Thiel, H. J. (1995). Classical swine fever virus: independent induction of protective immunity by two structural glycoproteins. *J. Virol.*, 69(10): 6479-6486.

[69] Stark R., Rümenapf T., Meyers G. and Thiel H. J. (1990). Genomic localization of hog cholera virus glycoproteins. *Virol.*, 174: 286-289.

[70] Mittelholzer, C., Moser, C., Tratschin, J. D. and Hofmann, M. A. (2000). Analysis of classical swine fever virus replication kinetics allows differentiation of highly virulent from avirulent strains. *Vet. Microbiol.*, 74(4): 293-308.

[71] Aoki, H., Ishikawa, K., Sakoda, Y., Sekiguchi, H., Kodama, M., Suzuki, S. and Fukusho, A., (2001). Characterization of classical swine fever virus associated with defective interfering particles containing a cytopathogenic subgenomic RNA isolated from wild boar. *J. Vet. Med. Sci.*, 63: 751-758.

[72] Fletcher, S. P. and Jackson, R. J. (2002). Pestivirus Internal Ribosome Entry Site (IRES) structure and function: Elements in the 5' untranslated region important for IRES function. *J. Virol.*, 76: 5024-5033.

[73] Kolupaeva, V. G., Pestova, T. V. and Hellen, C. U. (2000). Ribosomal binding to the internal ribosomal entry site of classical swine fever virus. RNA. 6: 1791-1807.

[74] Rijnbrand, R., van der, S. T., van Rijn, P. A., Spaan, W. J., Bredenbeek, P. J., 1997. Internal entry of ribosomes is directed by the 5' noncoding region of classical swine fever virus and is dependent on the presence of an RNA pseudoknot upstream of the initiation codon. *J. Virol.*, 71: 451-457.

[75] Lindenbach, B. D., and Rice, C. M. (2001). Flaviviridae: the viruses and their replication. In: D. M. Knipe, P. M. Howley, D. E. Griffin, R. A. Lamb, M. A. Martin, B. Roizman, S. E. Straus (Eds.), Fields Virology. Lippincott Williams & Wilkins, Philadelphia, pp. 991-1041.

[76] Rümenapf, T., Stark, R., Heimann, M. and Thiel, H. J. (1998). N-terminal protease of pestiviruses: identification of putative catalytic residues by site-directed mutagenesis. *J. Virol.*, 72: 2544-2547.

[77] Tratschin, J. D., Moser, C., Ruggli, N. and Hofmann, M. A. (1998). Classical swine fever virus leader proteinase Npro is not required for viral replication in cell culture. *J. Virol.*, 72: 7681-7684.

[78] Basler, C. F., Garcia-Sastre, A. (2002). Viruses and the type I interferon antiviral system: induction and evasion. *Int. Rev. Immunol.*, 21: 305– 337.

[79] Ruggli, N., Tratschin, J. D., Schweizer, M., McCullough, K. C., Hofmann, M. A. and Summerfield, A. (2003). Classical swine fever virus interferes with cellular antiviral defense: evidence for a novel function of Npro. *J. Virol.*, 77: 7645-7654.

[80] Ruggli, N., Bird, B. H., Liu, L., Bauhofer, O., Tratschin, J. D. and Hofmann, M. A. (2005). N^{pro} of classical swine fever virus is an antagonist of double-stranded RNA-mediated apoptosis and IFN-alpha/beta induction. Virology 340: 265-276.

[81] Hilton, L., Moganeradj, K., Zhang, G., Chen, Y. H., Randall, R. E., McCauley, J. W. and Goodbourn, S. (2006). The Npro product of bovine viral diarrhoea virus inhibits DNA binding by interferon regulatory factor 3 and targets it for proteasomal degradation. *J. Virol.*, 80: 11723-11732.

[82] La Rocca, S. A., Herbert, R. J., Crooke, H., Drew, T. W., Wileman, T. E. and Powell, P. P. (2005). Loss of interferon regulatory factor 3 in cells infected with classical swine fever virus involves the N-terminal protease, Npro. *J. Virol.*, 79: 7239-7247.

[83] Maniatis, T., Falvo, J. V., Kim, T. H., Kim, T. K., Lin, C. H., Parekh, B. S., Wathelet, M. G., 1998. Structure and function of the interferon-beta enhanceosome. *Cold Spring Harb. Symp. Quant. Biol.*, 63: 609-620.

[84] Merika, M. and Thanos, D. (2001). Enhanceosomes. *Curr. Opin. Genet. Dev.*, 11: 205-208.

[85] Rümenapf, T., Unger, G., Strauss, J. H. and Thiel, H. J. (1993). Processing of the envelope glycoproteins of pestiviruses. *J. Virol.*, 67: 3288-3294.

[86] Heimann, M., Roman-Sosa, G., Martoglio, B., Thiel, H. J., Rümenapf, T. (2006). Core protein of pestiviruses is processed at the C terminus by signal peptide peptidase. *J. Virol.*, 80: 1915-1921.

[87] Bruschke, C.J., Hulst, M.M., Moormann, R.J., van Rijn, P.A. and van Oirschot, J.T. (1997). Glycoprotein Erns of pestiviruses induces apoptosis in lymphocytes of several species. *J. Virol.*, 71: 6692-6696.

[88] Hausmann, Y., RomanSosa, G., Thiel, H. J. and Rümenapf, T. (2004). Classical swine fever virus glycoprotein E-rns is an endoribonuclease with an unusual base specificity. *J. Virol.*, 78: 5507-5512.

[89] Iqbal, M., Poole, E., Goodbourn, S. and McCauley, J. W. (2004). Role for bovine viral diarrhea virus Erns glycoprotein in the control of activation of beta interferon by double-stranded RNA. *J. Virol.*, 78: 136-145.

[90] Meyers, G., Ege, A., Fetzer, C., von, F.M., Elbers, K., Carr, V., Prentice, H., Charleston, B. and Schurmann, E. M. (2007). Bovine viral diarrhoea virus: Prevention of persistent foetal infection by a combination of two mutations affecting the Erns RNase and the Npro protease. *J. Virol.*, 81: 3327-3338.

[91] van Rijn, P. A., Miedema, G. K., Wensvoort, G., van Gennip, H. G. and Moormann, R. J. (1994). Antigenic structure of envelope glycoprotein E1 of hog cholera virus. *J. Virol.*, 68: 3934-3942.

[92] van Rijn, P. A., Bossers, A., Wensvoort, G. and Moormann, R. J. (1996). Classical swine fever virus (CSFV) envelope glycoprotein E2 containing one structural antigenic unit protects pigs from lethal CSFV challenge. *J. Gen. Virol.*, 77: 2737-2745.

[93] Harada, T., Tautz, N. and Thiel, H. J. (2000). E2-p7 region of the bovine viral diarrhea virus polyprotein: Processing and functional studies. *J. Virol.*, 74: 9498-9506.

[94] Pavlovic, D., Neville, D. C., Argaud, O., Blumberg, B., Dwek, R. A., Fischer, W. B. and Zitzmann, N. (2003). The hepatitis C virus p7 protein forms an ion channel that is inhibited by long-alkyl chain iminosugar derivatives. *Proc. Natl. Acad. Sci. U. S. A.*, 100: 6104-6108.

[95] Lackner, T., Muller, A., Pankraz, A., Becher, P., Thiel, H. J., Gorbalenya, A. E., Tautz, N. (2004). Temporal modulation of an autoprotease is crucial for replication and pathogenicity of an RNA virus. *J. Virol.*, 78: 10765-10775.

[96] Tautz, N., Elbers, K., Stoll, D., Meyers, G. and Thiel, H. J. (1997). Serine protease of pestiviruses: determination of cleavage sites. *J. Virol.*, 71: 5415-5422.

[97] Tautz, N., Kaiser, A. and Thiel, H. J. (2000). NS3 serine protease of bovine viral diarrhea virus: Characterization of active site residues, NS4A cofactor domain, and protease-cofactor interactions. *Virol.*, 273: 351-363.

[98] Xu, J., Mendez, E., Caron, P. R., Lin, C., Murcko, M. A., Collett, M. S. and Rice, C. M. (1997). Bovine viral diarrhea virus NS3 serine proteinase: polyprotein cleavage sites, cofactor requirements, and molecular model of an enzyme essential for pestivirus replication. *J. Virol.*, 71: 5312-5322.

[99] Lackner, T., Muller, A., Pankraz, A., Becher, P., Thiel, H. J., Gorbalenya, A. E. and Tautz, N. (2004). Temporal modulation of an autoprotease is crucial for replication and pathogenicity of an RNA virus. *J. Virol.*, 78: 10765-10775.

[100] Lackner, T., Muller, A., Konig, M., Thiel, H. J. and Tautz, N. (2005). Persistence of bovine viral diarrhea virus is determined by a cellular cofactor of a viral autoprotease. *J. Virol.*, 79: 9746-9755.

[101] Agapov, E. V., Murray, C. L., Frolov, I., Qu, L., Myers, T. M. and Rice, C. M. (2004). Uncleaved NS2-3 is required for production of infectious bovine viral diarrhea virus. *J. Virol.*, 78: 2414-2425.

[102] Moulin, H. R., Seuberlich, T., Bauhofer, O., Bennett, L. C., Tratschin, J. D., Hofmann, M. A. and Ruggli, N. (2007). Nonstructural proteins NS2-3 and NS4A of classical swine fever virus: essential features for infectious particle formation. Virology in press.

[103] Mackintosh, S. G., Lu, J. Z., Jordan, J. B., Harrison, M. K., Sikora, B., Sharma, S. D., Cameron, C. E., Raney, K. D. and Sakon, J. (2006). Structural and biological identification of residues on the surface of NS3 helicase required for optimal replication of the hepatitis C virus. *J. Biol. Chem.* 281: 3528-3535.

[104] Sampath, A., Xu, T., Chao, A., Luo, D., Lescar, J. and Vasudevan, S. G. (2006). Structure-based mutational analysis of the NS3 helicase from dengue virus. *J. Virol.*, 80: 6686-6690.

[105] Grassmann, C. W., Isken, O. and Behrens, S. E. (1999). Assignment of the multifunctional NS3 protein of bovine viral diarrhea virus during RNA replication: an in vivo and in vitro study. *J. Virol.*, 73: 9196-9205.

[106] Gu, B., Liu, C., Lin-Goerke, J., Maley, D. R., Gutshall, L. L., Feltenberger, C. A. and Del Vecchio, A. M. (2000). The RNA helicase and nucleotide triphosphatase activities of the bovine viral diarrhea virus NS3 protein are essential for viral replication. *J. Virol.*, 74: 1794-1800.

[107] Xu, J., Mendez, E., Caron, P. R., Lin, C., Murcko, M. A., Collett, M. S. and Rice, C. M. (1997). Bovine viral diarrhea virus NS3 serine proteinase: polyprotein cleavage sites, cofactor requirements, and molecular model of an enzyme essential for pestivirus replication. *J. Virol.*, 71(7): 5312-5322.

[108] Zhang, P., Xie, J., Yi, G., Zhang, C. and Zhou, R. (2005). De novo RNA synthesis and homology modeling of the classical swine fever virus RNA polymerase. *Virus Res.*, 112: 9-23.

[109] Grummer, B., Grotha, S. and Greiser-Wilke, I. (2004). Bovine viral diarrhoea virus is internalized by clathrin-dependent receptor-mediated endocytosis. *J. Vet. Med. B Infect. Dis. Vet. Public Health.*, 51: 427-432.

[110] Krey, T., Thiel, H. J. and Rümenapf, T. (2005). Acid-resistant bovine pestivirus requires activation for pH-triggered fusion during entry. *J. Virol.,* 79: 4191-4200.

[111] Krey, T., Moussay, E., Thiel, H. J. and Rümenapf, T. (2006). Role of the low-density lipoprotein receptor in entry of bovine viral diarrhea virus. *J. Virol.,* 80: 10862-10867.

[112] Maurer, K., Krey, T., Moennig, V., Thiel, H. R. and Rümenapf, T. (2004). CD46 is a cellular receptor for bovine viral diarrhea virus. *J. Virol.,* 78: 1792-1799.

[113] Hulst, M. M. and Moormann, R. J. (1997). Inhibition of pestivirus infection in cell culture by envelope proteins E (rns) and E2 of classical swine fever virus: E (rns) and E2 interact with different receptors. *J. Gen. Virol.,* 78: 2779-2787.

[114] Wang, Z., Nie, Y. C., Wang, P. G., Ding, M. X., and Deng, H. K. (2004). Characterization of classical swine fever virus entry by using pseudotyped viruses: E1 and E2 are sufficient to mediate viral entry. *Virol.,* 330: 332-341.

[115] Quinkert, D., Bartenschlager, R. and Lohmann, V. (2005). Quantitative analysis of the hepatitis C virus replication complex. *J. Virol.,* 79: 13594-13605.

[116] Salonen, A., Ahola, T. and Kaariainen, L. (2005). Viral RNA replication in association with cellular membranes. *Curr. Top. Microbiol. Immunol.,* 285: 139-173.

[117] Westaway, E. G., Mackenzie, J. M. and Khromykh, A. A. (2003). Kunjin RNA replication and applications of Kunjin replicons. *Adv. Virus Res.,* 59: 99-140.

[118] Moulin, H. R., Seuberlich, T., Bauhofer, O., Bennett, L. C., Tratschin, J. D., Hofmann, M. A. and Ruggli, N. (2007). Nonstructural proteins NS2-3 and NS4A of classical swine fever virus: essential features for infectious particle formation. *Virol.,* in press.

[119] Hu¨gle, T., F. Fehrmann, E., B., Kohara, M., Krausslich, H. G., Rice, C. M., Blum, H. E. Moradpour, D. (2001). The hepatitis C virus non-structural protein 4B is an integral endoplasmic reticulum membrane protein. *Virol.,* 284: 70–81.

[120] Lundin, M., Lindstrom, H., Gronwall, C. and Persson, M. A. (2006). Dual topology of the processed hepatitis C virus protein NS4B is influenced by the NS5A protein. *J. Gen. Virol.,* 87: 3263–3272.

[121] Lundin, M., Monne, M., Widell, A., Von Heijne, G. and Persson, M. A. (2003). Topology of the membrane-associated hepatitis C virus protein NS4B. *J. Virol.,* 77: 5428–5438.

[122] Qu, L., McMullan, L. K. and Rice, C. M. (2001). Isolation and characterization of noncytopathic pestivirus mutants reveals a role for nonstructural protein NS4B in viral cytopathogenicity. *J. Virol.,* 75: 10651–10662.

[123] Fernandez-Sainz, D. P., Gladue, L. G., Holinka, L. G., O'Donnell, V., Gudmundsdottir, I., Prarat, M. V., Patch, J. R., Golde, W. T., Lu, Z., Zhu, J., Carrillo, C., Risatti, G. R. and Borca, M. V. (2010). Mutations in Classical Swine Fever Virus NS4B affect virulence in swine. *J. Virol.,* 84(3): 1536-1549.

[124] Lai, V. C. H., Zhong, W. D., Skelton, A., Ingravallo, P., Vassilev, V., Donis, R. O., Hong, Z., Lau, J. Y. N. (2000). Generation and characterization of a hepatitis C virus NS3 protease-dependent bovine viral diarrhea virus. *J. Virol.,* 74: 6339–6347.

[125] Rumenapf, T., Stark, R., Heimann, M. and Thiel, H. J. (1998). N-terminal protease of pestiviruses: identification of putative catalytic residues by site directed mutagenesis. *J. Virol.,* 72: 2544–2547.

[126] Stark, R., Meyers, G., Rumenapf, T. and Thiel, H. J. (1993). Processing of pestivirus polyprotein: cleavage site between autoprotease and nucleocapsid protein of classical swine fever virus. *J. Virol.*, 67: 7088–7095.

[127] Zhou, A., Paranjape, J. M., Der, S. D., Williams, B. R. and Silverman, R. H. (1999). Interferon action in triply deficient mice reveals the existence of alternative antiviral pathways. *Virol.*, 258: 435–440.

[128] Roehe, P. M., Woodward, M. J. and Edwards, S. (1992). Characterisation of p20 gene sequences from a border disease-like pestivirus isolated from pigs. *Vet. Microbiol.*, 33: 231-238.

[129] Ruggli, N., Tratshin, J.D., Schweizer, M., McCullough, K.C., Hofmann, M.A. and Summerfield, A. (2003). Classical Swine Fever Virus interferes with Cellular Antiviral Defense: Evidence for a Novel Function of N^{pro}. *J. Virol.*, 77: 7645-7654.

[130] Chandranaik, B. M., Renukaprasad, C., Patil, S. S, Venkatesha, M. D, Giridhar, P, Byregowda, S. M and Prabhudas, K. (2011). Development of cell culture based inactivated Classical swine fever vaccine. *Ind. Vet. J.*, 88 (4): 16–18.

[131] Summerfield, A., Hofmann, M. A. & McCullough, K. C. (1998a). Low density blood granulocytic cells induced during classical swine fever are targets for virus infection. *Vet. Immunol. Immunopathol.*, 63: 289–301.

[132] Ambagala, A.P., Solheim, J.C. and Srikumaran, S. (2005). Viral interference with MHC class I antigen presentation pathway: the battle continues. *Vet. Immunol. Immunopathol.*, 107: 1-15.

[133] Schweizer, M. & Peterhans, E. (2001). Noncytopathic bovine viral diarrhea virus inhibits double-stranded RNA-induced apoptosis and interferon synthesis. *J. Virol.*, 75: 4692–4698.

[134] Baigent, S. J., Zhang, G., Fray, M.D., Flick-Smith, H., Goodbourn, S. and J. W. McCauley. (2002). Inhibition of beta interferon transcription by non-cytopathogenic bovine viral diarrhea virus is through an interferon regulatory factor 3-dependent mechanism. *J. Virol.*, 76: 8979–8988.

[135] Knoetig, S. M., Summerfield, A., Spagnuolo-Weaver, M. and McCullough, K.C. (1999). Immunopathogenesis of classical swine fever: role of monocytic cells. *Immunol.*, 97: 359–366.

[136] Banchereau, J., Briere, F., Caux, C., Davoust, J., Lebecque, S., Liu, Y. J., Pulendran, B. and Palucka, K. (2000). Immunobiology of dendritic cells. *Annu. Rev. Immunol.*, 18: 767–811.

[137] Steinman, R. M. (1991). The dendritic cell system and its role in immunogenicity. *Annu. Rev. Immunol.*, 9: 271–296.

[138] Pulendran, B., Palucka, K. and Banchereau, J. (2001). Sensing pathogens and tuning immune responses. *Sci.*, 293: 253–256.

[139] Van Oirschot, J. T., De Jong, D. & Huffels, N. D. (1983). Effect of infections with swine fever virus on immune functions. II. Lymphocyte response to mitogens and enumeration of lymphocyte subpopulations. *Vet. Microbiol.*, 8: 81–95.

[140] Steinman, R. M. (1991). The dendritic cell system and its role in immunogenicity. *Annu. Rev. Immunol.*, 9: 271–296.

[141] Summerfield, A., Guzylack-Piriou, L., Schaub, A., Carrasco, C. P. Tache, V. & Charley, B. (2003). Porcine peripheral blood dendritic cells and natural interferon-producing cells. *Immunol.*, 110: 440–449.

[142] Trautwein, G. (1988). Pathology and pathogenesis of the disease. In Classical Swine Fever and Related Infections, pp. 27–54. Edited by B. Liess. Boston: Martinus Nijhoff Publishing.

[143] McCullough, K. C., Ruggli, N. and Summerfield, A. (2009). Dendritic cells – At the front-line of pathogen attack. *Vet. Immunol. Sympos.*, 128(1-3): 7-15.

[144] Bauhofer, O., Summerfield, A., McCullough, K. C. and Ruggli, N. (2005). Role of double-stranded RNA and N^{pro} of classical swine fever virus in the activation of monocyte-derived dendritic cells. *Virol.*, 343(1): 93-105.

[145] Horscroft, N., Bellows, D., Ansari, I., Lai, V. C., Dempsey, S., Liang, D., Donis, R., Zhong, W. and Hong, Z. (2005). Establishment of a sub genomic replicon for bovine viral diarrhoea virus in Huh-7 cells and modulation of interferon-regulated factor 3-mediated antiviral response. *J. Virol.*, 79: 2788– 2796.

[146] Carrasco, C. P., Rigden, R. C., Vincent, I. E., Balmelli, C., Ceppi, M., Bauhofer, O., Tache, V., Hjertner, B., McNeilly, F., van Gennip, H. G., McCullough, K. C. and Summerfield, A. (2004). Interaction of classical swine fever virus with dendritic cells. *J. Gen. Virol.*, 85: 1633-1641.

[147] Ressang, A. A. (1973). Studies on the pathogenesis of hog cholera. II. Virus distribution in tissue and the morphology of the immune response. *Zentbl. Vetmed. Reihe.*, 20: 272–288.

[148] Cella, M., Salio, M., Sakakibara, Y., Langen, H., Julkunen, I. & Lanzavecchia, A. (1999). Maturation, activation, and protection of dendritic cells induced by double-stranded RNA. *J. Exp. Med.*, 189: 821–829.

[149] Gomez-Villamandos, J. C., Salguero, F. J., Ruiz-Villamor, E., Sanchez-Cordon, P. J., Bautista, M. J. & Sierra, M. A. (2003). Classical swine fever: pathology of bone marrow. *Vet. Pathol.*, 40: 157–163.

[150] Lackner, T., Muller, A., Pankraz, A., Becher, P., Thiel, H.J., Gorbalenya, A.E. and Tautz, N. (2004). Temporal modulation of an autoprotease is crucial for replication and pathogenicity of an RNA virus. *J. Virol.*, 78: 10765– 10775.

[151] Iqbal, M., Poole, E., Goodbourn, S. and McCauley, J.W. (2004). Role for bovine viral diarrhea virus E^{rns} glycoprotein in the control of activation of beta interferon by double-stranded RNA. *J. Virol.*, 78: 136– 145.

[152] Wang, C. S., Chen, S. C., Yu, N. J., Chien, M. S., Lin, C. C. and Lee, W. C. The Down-regulation of MHC molecule of monocytic cells after classical swine fever virus infection. Graudte Institute of Veterinary Pathology and Department of Veterinary Medicine, National Chung Hsing University, Taiwan, ROC.

[153] Murphy, F. A., Gibbs, E. P. J., Horzinek, M. C. and Studdert, M. J. Veterinary Virology, 3rd Edition.

[154] Susa, M., Konig, M., Saalmuller, A., Reddehase, M. J. and Thiel, H. J. (1992). Pathogenesis of Classical Swine Fever: B-lymphocyte deficiency caused caused by Hog cholera virus. *J. Virol.*, 66(2): 1171-1175.

[155] Gallagher, R. B., and Osmond, D. G. (1991). To B, or not to B: that is the question. Immunol. Today. 12: 1-3.

[156] Ehrensperger, F. (1989). Immunological aspects of the infection, p. 143-163. In B. Liess (ed.), Classical swine fever and related viral infections. Martinus Nijhoff Publishing, Boston.

[157] Van Oirschot, J. T. (1988). Description of the virus infection, p. 1-25. In B. Liess (ed.), Classical swine fever and related viral infections. Martinus Nijhoff Publishing, Boston.

Chapter 5

Viral Replication Strategies: Manipulation of ER Stress Response Pathways and Promotion of IRES-Dependent Translation

Paul J. Hanson, Huifang M. Zhang, Maged Gomaa Hemida,
Xin Ye, Ye Qiu and Decheng Yang

Additional information is available at the end of the chapter

http://dx.doi.org/10.5772/56072

1. Introduction

Translation initiation is a rate-limiting step of protein synthesis. Therefore, it is highly regulated by different mechanisms, which depend upon the structural characteristics of a given mRNA. Most cellular mRNAs are translated by a cap-dependent mechanism that requires the binding of the trimeric complex of eukaryotic initiation factors (eIF)4F, comprised of eIF4G, eIF4E and eIF4A, to the 7-methyl GpppN cap structure at the 5′ end of the mRNA. However, many viral and some cellular mRNAs have evolved a cap-independent mechanism of translation initiation that uses a highly structured internal ribosome-entry site (IRES) sequence located in the 5′ untranslated region (5′UTR) of their mRNA (Holcik & Sonenberg, 2005). The IRES was first discovered in poliovirus (a typical member of picornaviruses) and later in other viruses such as hepatitis C virus (HCV), HIV, Herpesviruses, etc., and also in many cellular mRNAs (Jang, et al., 1988, Labadie, et al., 2004, Locker, et al., 2011, Pelletier & Sonenberg, 1988). Cellular physiological conditions dictate when a given mRNA uses cap-dependent or IRES-dependent translation initiation. Under normal conditions, cellular mRNAs translation is initiated by a cap-dependent mechanism; however, under stress conditions, such as starvation, irradiation, heat shock, hypoxia, toxin and viral infection, the translation initiation is switched from cap-dependent to an IRES-driven mechanism, which may be on the same mRNA (Komar & Hatzoglou, 2005, Spriggs, et al., 2005).

Several viral infections trigger endoplasmic reticulum (ER) stress responses in a variety of ways inside the host cell. One of the most significant effects is the shutting off of global, cap-dependent translation, which results in activation of IRES-dependent translational mechanisms. This is quite apparent in picornaviruses because their viral mRNA does not contain a cap structure at the 5'end. Also, its IRES located in the 5'UTR recruits ribosomes and other factors, which then scan to reach the initiation codon without the requirement of the eIF4E (Jang, et al., 2009, Jang, 2006). IRES containing viruses are able to benefit from the ER stress response, enhancing their own protein synthesis while also enhancing their self-defense capability. There are several mechanisms by which virus infections and other stress signals achieve inhibition of cap-dependent translation of cellular mRNAs, including: i) site specific cleavage of cellular translational initiation factors, such as the eukaryotic translation initiation factor 4GI (eIF4GI) by picornaviral and HIV proteases (Chau, et al., 2007, Etchison, et al., 1982, Lamphear, et al., 1993, Ohlmann, et al., 2002) or by cellular caspases (Marissen & Lloyd, 1998). ii) phosphorylation of eIF2α and other co-factors of translation. The site specific cleavage or modification of translation factors does not affect IRES-driven translation, but instead promotes IRES-containing mRNA to utilize the cleaved translation initiation factor or specific IRES transacting factors (ITAFs) for their translation (Morley, et al., 2005, Raught, 2007). (iii) overproduction of homologous proteins of cap-binding protein eIF4E (e.g. 4E-BP), which compete with eIF4G limiting its binding (Marcotrigiano, et al., 1999) to eIF4E iv) suppression of eIF4E expression by certain microRNAs (Ho, et al., 2011, Mathonnet, et al., 2007).

The rapid inhibition of cellular cap-dependent protein synthesis has been demonstrated as a critical precursor to cell fate. In this context, it is noteworthy that the IRES-containing cellular mRNAs are found to be preferentially involved in the control of cell fate by functioning to promote cell growth and survival or apoptosis (Jackson, et al., 2010, Sonenberg & Hinnebusch, 2009, Spriggs, et al., 2005). Notable genes include the B-cell lymphoma-2 (Bcl-2) family proteins, apoptotic protease activating factor 1 (Apaf-1), checkpoint homolog kinase 1(chk-1), eIF4GII, p53 and 78kDa Glucose-regulated protein 78 or Binding immunoglobulin protein (GRP78/BiP) (Komar, et al., 2005, Spriggs, et al., 2005). It was therefore suggested that IRES-mediated translation plays a critical role in regulation of cell fate (Spriggs, et al., 2005). Cellular genes containing IRESs in their mRNA are continually being discovered, some amid controversy as being true IRESs (Shatsky, et al., 2010). Previous studies have indicated that the cell fate decision is made based on the severity and duration of the stress signal. Under a transient stress or during the early phase of infection, the IRES will mediate translation initiation of genes promoting cell survival/growth, which enhance cellular capability to combat viral infection. However, under a severe or prolonged stress such as persistent infection of picornaviruses, translation initiation will selectively express the genes responsible for inducing cell apoptosis (Henis-Korenblit, et al., 2002, Lewis, et al., 2008), effectively destroying the host cells and potentially limiting the viral infection of surrounding cells. In any circumstance, the host cell will employ an alternate way to defend itself. In this chapter, we will discuss the recent advances in the understanding of IRES-mediated translational control of genes under stress conditions, with a particular focus on ER stress caused by picornaviral and other viral infections.

2. Viral Manipulation of ER stress pathways and components

The ER stress response or unfolded protein response (UPR) is a major component of disease (Tabas & Ron, 2011). Many viral infections induce ER stress and have adapted mechanisms to modulate the stress response and its effectors. On the cellular level, ER stress may be triggered by many factors, including serum starvation, hypoxia, changes in calcium homeostasis, viral infections, as well as other perturbations (Chakrabarti, et al., 2011). In general, ER stress is triggered by the accumulation of misfolded or unfolded proteins in the ER lumen. In response to this stress, a coordinated adaptive program termed the unfolded protein response (UPR) is activated and serves to minimize the accumulation and aggregation of misfolded proteins (Chakrabarti, et al., 2011). The molecules and signaling pathways of the UPR may vary slightly dependent upon cell type. The stress response or UPR is regulated by master regulatory protein, BiP or GRP78. The initial, transient phase of the ER stress response functions to increase the removal or degradation and folding of misfolded or unfolded proteins. In its non-stressed state, BiP is bound to the ER luminal domain of the transmembrane proteins including PKR-like ER kinase (PERK), inositol requiring enzyme 1 (IRE1) and activating transcription factor 6 (ATF6) (Chakrabarti, et al., 2011). These are the three major arms of the UPR. Viral infection causes the rapid accumulation of viral and other cellular proteins trafficked to the ER. When excess proteins accumulate in the ER lumen, BiP dissociates from its three transmembrane sensors, resulting in the functional activation of the 3 major arms of the UPR. PERK and IRE1 are activated and undergo homodimerization and auto-phosphorylation (Bollo, et al., 2010, Liu, et al., 2000, Oikawa & Kimata, 2010), triggering their downstream genes. The activation of the IRE1 pathway leads to the splicing of X box binding protein 1 (XBP-1) (Lee, et al., 2002). This spliced form of XBP-1 mRNA encodes an active transcription factor that binds to the promoter of unfold protein response element (UPRE) to induce expression of a subset of genes encoding protein degradation enzymes, resulting in ER-associated misfolded protein degradation (Lee, et al., 2003). The activation of PERK results in the phosphorylation of eIF2 on its α subunit (Raven & Koromilas, 2008). eIF2α phosphorylation effectively shuts down global, cap-dependent protein synthesis and causes a shift in translation to that of cellular mRNA containing IRESs reducing the burden of accumulating proteins in the ER (Harding, et al., 2002). This constitutes a translational switch to IRES-mediated translation initiation. UPR activation also involves the trafficking of ATF6 by BiP, resulting in its migration to the Golgi apparatus, where it is cleaved by S1P and S2P proteases, releasing a soluble fragment that enters the nucleus and bind to promoters containing the ER stress response elements (ERSE) and ATF/cAMP response elements (CREs) to activate ER chaperone genes, such as BiP, GRP94, and calreticulin (Yoshida, et al., 2001). These newly synthesized chaperones refold misfolded proteins in the ER in an effort to relieve ER stress. ATF6 also promotes XBP1 splicing (Lee, et al., 2002), indicating the interconnectedness of the three branches of the UPR. The shift from cap-dependent to cap-independent translation mediated by ER stress is critical to both cell fate and viral infection productivity. Many viruses, particularly RNA viruses, such as members of the *Picornaviridae* family, have evolved to replicate through cap-independent mechanisms, thus the shut-off of global protein synthesis induced by ER stress is of major strategic importance.

When ER stress is chronic or prolonged, it leads to the induction of ER mediated apoptosis (Tabas, et al., 2011). As is the case in viral infection, viral proteases also inhibit select cellular translational components, which may be initiated by ER stress. Our group has demonstrated that CVB3 protease 2A and 3C can cleave eIFGI and induce cell apoptosis (Chau, et al., 2007). Viral proteins, such as picornaviral protein 2B, have been shown to contribute to the depletion of calcium stores within the ER (Wang, et al., 2010), furthering the viral life cycle by contributing to viral release. Prolonged and sustained severe ER stress eventually drives the cell to apoptosis (Mekahli, et al., 2011). Although significant progress in our understanding of apoptosis initiated by ER stress has been made in recent years, the molecular mechanisms of ER induced apoptosis are yet to be fully elucidated. During prolonged/severe ER stress, the functions of the three branches of the UPR (IRE1, ATF-6 and PERK) act in concert during prolonged/severe ER stress to induce apoptosis. Under those conditions, the endonuclease activity of IRE1 becomes less specific. As a result IRE1 contributes to the degradation of membrane associated mRNA, termed regulated IRE1 dependent degradation (RIDD). RIDD activation and XBP1 splicing highlight the two distinct functions for IRE1 during ER stress, the former being apoptotic and the latter generally regarded as protective (Hollien, et al., 2009). Previous studies indicate a correlation between enhanced ER stress induced apoptosis and the induction of RIDD activity. RIDD activation requires the nuclease domain of IRE1 to be activated, whereas IRE1 induced XBP1 splicing is modulated by IRE1 kinase domain activation (Hollien, et al., 2009). IRE1 has also been shown to bind Bcl-2 homologous antagonist/killer (Bak) and Bcl-2 associated x protein (Bax) (Hetz, et al., 2006), two pro-apoptotic proteins from the Bcl-2 family previously described in mitochondria derived apoptosis. Recently, however, it was shown that Bax translocates not only to the mitochondria, but also to the ER membrane during prolonged ER stress (Gotoh, et al., 2004, Hetz, et al., 2006, McCullough, et al., 2001, Wang, et al., 2010). Once translocated to the ER membrane, Bax permeabilizes the membrane, causing ER luminal proteins to be translocated to the cytosol (Wang, et al., 2010). Normally anti-apoptotic in function, BiP, once in the cytoplasm translocates to the plasma membrane where it becomes an apoptotic inducing receptor for prostate apoptosis response-4 (Par-4) (Wang, et al., 2010). Par-4 has been shown to co-localize with BiP in the ER. The binding of Par-4 to membrane bound BiP activates the extrinsic apoptotic cascade through FADD, caspase8 and caspase3 (Burikhanov, et al., 2009). Interestingly, the secretion of Par-4 is activated by TRAIL (Hart & El-Deiry, 2009). Several viruses including avian H5N1 and HIV have been shown promote cell death through TRAIL activated apoptosis in macrophages by enhancing TRAIL induced caspase10 activation (Ekchariyawat, et al., 2011, Zhu, et al., 2011).

Additionally, during prolonged and severe ER stress, PERK also enhances the translation of specific downstream genes, including ATF-4 (activating transcription factor-4) (Fels & Koumenis, 2006). ATF-4 is able to activate pro-apoptotic C/EBP homologous protein (CHOP) during conditions of prolonged, severe ER stress (Ma, et al., 2002). CHOP acts to induce apoptosis by promoting constitutively expressed Bax translocation to the mithochondria through inhibition of anti-apoptotic Bcl-2 transcription, as Bcl-2 functions to inhibit Bax in pro-survival conditions (Gotoh, et al., 2004, McCullough, et al., 2001). Here we see a connection between apoptosis mediated by IRE1 (by binding to Bax/Bak) and by PERK-mediated CHOP activation through ATF4, stressing the importance of cross talk between the three arms of the UPR. Interestingly, CHOP acts as a negative regulator of eIF2α phosphorylation as well

(Novoa, et al., 2001). The importance of the pathways described above in both global translation attenuation and apoptosis has made them the target of manipulation of many viruses. For example, Hepatitis E virus (HEV) open reading frame 2 protein (ORF-2) is able to modulate ER stress induced apoptosis by increasing eIF2α phosphorylation and activation of CHOP, simultaneously (John, et al., 2011). Our lab also obtained a similar result in studying coxsackievirus B3 (CVB3)-induced apoptosis through phosphorylation of eIF2α and activation of CHOP; however, this activation is not through ATF4 but through ATF6 (Zhang, et al., 2010). For HEV, during infection, CHOP, which normally induces apoptosis and translocation of Bax to the mitochondria, is unable to perform this pro-apoptotic function. This is due to the simultaneous activation and interaction of heat-shock proteins Hsp-70B, Hsp-72 and Hsp-40 by HEV protein ORF-2 (John, et al., 2011). Several members of the heat shock protein family, including Hsp-70, have been demonstrated to contain an IRES element in its long 5′UTR region of mRNA (Ahmed & Duncan, 2004, Hernandez, et al., 2004). This strategic modulation of pro-apoptosis and pro-survival proteins occurs presumably to delay apoptosis, while allowing the viral replication cycle to continue to completion. This demonstrates the careful strategic interplay between the virus and host translational factors as well as host cell components of the UPR. In doing so, a given virus is able to modulate the delicate balance between apoptosis and survival.

3. Structures of IRES

3.1. Classification of viral IRESs

IRES dependent translation initiation was first described in 1988 in the 5′UTR of the RNA genome of poliovirus (PV) (Pelletier, et al., 1988). Since this original discovery, IRES elements have been identified in the long, highly structured 5′UTR of almost all picornaviruses, including encephalomyocarditis virus (EMCV) (Lindeberg & Ebendal, 1999), Foot-and-mouth disease virus (FMDV) (Ohlmann&Jackson, 1999), Coxsackievirus B3 (Yang, et al., 1997) human rhinoviruses (HRV) (Rojas-Eisenring, et al., 1995), and other viruses, such as, Hepatitis A(Ali, et al., 2001), HIV (Weill, et al., 2009) and DNA viruses such as Kaposi's sarcoma-associated herpesvirus (KSHV) (Bieleski,, et al., 2004). Inherit to viral strategy, viruses must hijack cellular translational machinery, facilitating their own translation and replication. Translation initiation is the rate-limiting step of translation, which is the reason that it has evolved as a key strategic process, vital to viral strategy. Picornaviral mRNA, like many RNA viruses, is uncapped or lacks the 5′ terminal m^7GpppN cap structure found in cellular mRNAs (Belsham, 2009). Instead, picornaviruses and other IRES translating viruses contain a small, virus-encoded peptide or VPg (Jang, et al., 1990). The discovery of IRES elements across a variety of viruses also identified distinct structural and functional differences amongst them, leading to the implementation of an IRES classification scheme. Viral IRESs are subdivided into four categories based on their structure, function and mechanism of initiation of translation. All four IRES types commonly share the necessity of (on some level) involving non-canonical translational factors that interact with IRES and replace the function of some canonical translation initiation factors. The canonical translation factors involved also vary dependent upon the IRES structure, degree of interaction, and form the basis for IRES designation and classification.

3.2. Type I IRESs

Type I IRESs (fig.1) comprise enteroviruses and rhinoviruses. These IRESs contain a tetra-loop, cloverleaf structure in stem loop position I that resembles the 4-way junction of tRNA. This structure interacts with host cellular protein poly(rC)-binding protein 2 (PCBP2) and viral protein 3CD to form a bridge between the 5′ and 3′ ends to facilitate multiple rounds of viral replication (Fernandez-Miragall, et al., 2009). Downstream of the cloverleaf stem loop at position I are three distinctive C-rich motifs that precede the stem loop at position II. Two more C-rich regions are present in domain IV. There is also a pyrimidine tract motif located downstream of domain V, with a silent AUG region found 10-15 bases further downstream.

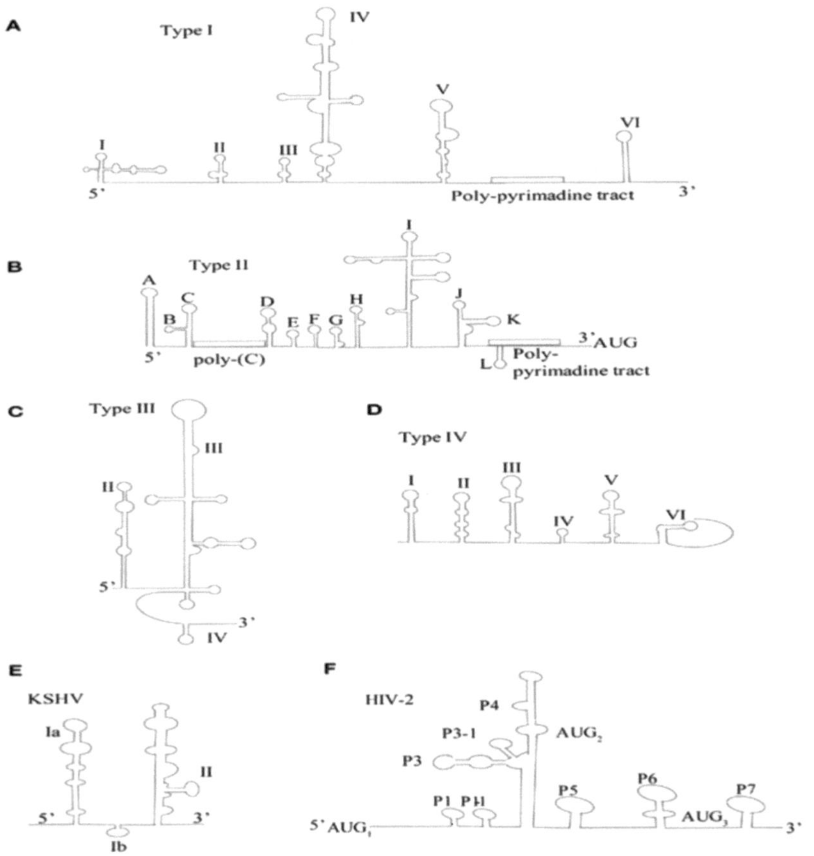

Figure 1. Schematic of proposed secondary structure of viral IRESs. A) Type I IRES represented by PV-1 (adapted from Jang, 2006) B) Type II IRES represented by EMCV (adapted from Jang,, 2006) C) Type III IRES represented by HCV (adapted from Beales, 2003 D) Type IV IRES represented by Plautia stali intestine virus (PSIV) (adapted from Kanamori, and Nakashima, 2001) E) DNA virus IRES represented by Kaposi's sarcoma-associated herpesvirus (KSHV) (adapted from Beales, 2003) F) HIV IRES, represent by HIV-2 (adapted from Locker, 2010)

The functional AUG initiation codon is traditionally further downstream from the silent AUG in type I IRESs, so the ribosome must scan downstream to the next AUG to begin translation initiation. Type I IRESs contain an eIF4G binding site that is absent the N-terminal region. This is due to viral protease cleavage of eIF4G to produce a truncated, yet functional form. This truncation eliminates its N-terminal region that contains a cap-binding domain. It is this feature that allows the ribosome to be recruited independent of the cap-structure, which is the hallmark of IRES-dependent translation. N-terminal deficient eIF4G is the integral translation initiation factor in the recruitment of the 43S ribosomal subunit, a process that is further enhanced by eIF4A. In fact, mutations made to the eIF4G-binding domain of the poliovirus IRES are the basis for the mutation of the PV strain given as the vaccine, further stressing the importance of translation initiation as a rate-limiting step (Malnou, et al., 2004). All together, type I IRESs contain six stem loops termed stem loops I-VI. The authentic IRES structure is located in the stem loop II-VI region, which facilitates initiation and translation of the viral genome (Pelletier, et al., 1988). Many of the canonical translation initiation factors, with the exception of eIF4E and the N-terminal region of eIF4G, are necessary for type I and II IRES translation. For this reason, viral modulation of these cap-dependent translation initiation factors has been identified as a vital component to viral strategy. Type I and II IRESs also utilize non-canonical translation initiation factors, termed IRES-specific cellular transacting factors (ITAFs). Examples of ITAFs include La autoantigen, PTB (pyrimidine tract binding protein) and UNR (upstream of N-Ras) (Costa-Mattioli, et al., 2004, Verma, et al., 2010, Cornelis, et al., 2005). ITAFs allow for the bypass of canonical translation initiation factors that are likely functionally inhibited and the target of viral strategy, either through direct proteolytic cleavage or modulation of pathways (such as UPR modulation).

3.3. Type II IRESs

Type II IRESs (fig.1) comprise the cardio- and apthoviruses of the *Picornavirdiae* family. There are several features of the IRES structure which differentiates the type II from that of the type I IRES. The 5'UTR are significantly longer than their type I counterparts. In place of the cloverleaf structure at stem loop position I, there is a hairpin or S structure. Just downstream of the S structure is an ~200bp C-tract that separates the S structure from the coding region. In between the C rich tract and the coding region there are three structural distinct regions. The first are 2 to 4 pseudoknots, next is the cis-acting replication element (cre) and lastly the IRES element, which spans stem loops II-V, also termed H-L. Just downstream are two AUG triplets that actively initiate protein synthesis. Interestingly, each produces a unique version of the leader protein. Type II IRESs require many of the canonical translation initiation factors. eIF4G, eIF4A and eIF4B have been demonstrated to interact with the SL J/K/L regions of the type II IRESs, with mutations to these domains causing reductions in IRES activity (Jang, 2006). As mentioned above, viral IRESs often utilize ITAFs, which further enhance translation in the absence of the canonical translation factors. The variability of ITAFs and canonical translation factors seen amongst the four types of IRESs is indicative of differences amongst IRES structural components, which are able mimic the function of both.

3.4. Type III IRES

Type III IRES (fig.1) structures demonstrate a new level of IRES-mediated translation initiation in which they are able to induce conformational changes directly to the ribosome that influence its entry, position and stability (Hellen, 2009). Flaviviruses, such as hepatitis C virus (HCV), contain IRESs considered to be prototypical of type III IRESs. The HCV IRES contains 3 distinctive domains, II, III and IV. Domain II is an irregular shaped, long stem loop structure. Domain III is a pseudoknot that also contains several hairpin-structured sub-domains, IIIa-IIIf, whereas domain IV is a short hairpin structure containing the initiation codon. The HCV IRES, like all other type III IRESs, is able to directly and independently bind the 40S subunit, thereby bypassing the need for canonical eIFs 4A, 4B, 4F, 1 and 1A. Hepatitis C virus (HCV) has been shown to require eIF3 and the eIF2•GTP/Met-tRNA$^{Met}{}_{i}$. ternary complex to bind sequentially for translation initiation. However, some type III IRESs, such as the Simian picornavirus type 9 (SPV9) IRES, have been shown to promote Met-tRNA$^{Met}{}_{i}$ recruitment to the ribosome independent of eIF2 (de Breyne, et al., 2008). Therefore negating the need for eIF2, which is quite often phosphorylated (i.e. translationally inactivated) during viral infection due to interferon activation of PKR or PERK, which induce subsequent phosphorylation of the eIF2α subunit. Type III IRES-containing viral mRNA has been demonstrated to be more resistant to translation inhibition caused by eIF2α phosphorylation than that of the cap-dependent cellular mRNAs (Pestova, et al., 2008).

3.5. Type IV IRES

Type IV IRESs (fig.2) initiate translation on the intergenic region (IGR) by direct binding of the 40S subunit or to the 80S ribosome. They are represented by the dicistroviruses, particularly the cricket paralysis virus (CrPV), which contain the smallest regions for internal ribosomal entry. Structurally, its IRES consists of 3 distinct domains. Each domain contains a pseudoknot and may or may not contain a hairpin like structure in stem loop 3. Type IV IRESs translation initiation occurs without involving any canonical initiation factors, initiator tRNA, or a proper AUG start codon. In contrast to conventional AUG codon for IRES translation initiation, the start codon of type IV IRESs may be GCU, GCA, GCC or CAA. In fact, studies have shown that translation initiation of CrPV IRES is impaired by the promotion of the eIF2•GTP/Met-tRNA$^{Met}{}_{i}$.ternary complex to the 40S subunit. This may be an evolutionary advancement of conditions where the eIF2α is phosphorylated, such as during ER stress and viral infection (Hellen, 2009).

3.6. IRES of Lentiviruses

The HIV IRESs (fig.1) represent yet another new class of IRES, not previously characterized by the four IRES types already described. On one hand, it displays type III IRES properties possessing the ability to directly and indirectly bind to 40s and eIF3 (Locker, et al., 2011). On the other hand, it requires all eIF's except for eIF4E and eIF1, a property of class I and II IRESs (Locker, et al., 2010). The structure of the HIV IRES is highly complex. It contains a long 5′UTR harboring a Tar stem loop, Poly-A, PBS, DIS, SD and Psi regions (Vallejos, et al., 2011). Interestingly, in contrast to its type I, II and III IRES counterparts, the HIV IRES appears to be resistant to structural mutations which to date have been unable to alter its function (Vallejos, et al., 2011). Also unique is its ability to recruit three initiation complexes to a single RNA molecule (Locker, et al., 2010). The translational requirements of HIV IRESs lend themselves to the notion that, while able to be translated cap-dependently, HIV RNA possesses and indeed utilizes IRESs as part of a tightly regulated and conserved method of cap-independent translation. The redundant ability of HIV to translate through a variety of mechanisms highlights the importance of translation being a key, highly regulated process of the viral lifecycle. The utilization of the HIV IRESs takes place relatively late in the viral life cycle and is regulated by the G2/M phase of the cell cycle, also activated by osmotic stress (Vallejos, et al., 2011). This is particularly interesting given that cap-dependent translation is shut-off during the cell cycle, leading to the notion of a new level of evolutionary complexity exemplified by the ability of HIV to modulate translation between cap-dependent and independent translation based on cell physiology. The HIV IRES also utilizes a subset of ITAFs that are exclusively available during the G2/M phase (Vallejos, et al., 2011). The utilization of its IRES is thought to regulate the transition between translation and encapsidation. The HIV-2 virus is only able to be encapsidated once the cognate form of it is translated, versus HIV-1 that can be either translated or propagated as a genome and encapsidated into virons (Locker, et al., 2010). This is suggestive of a possible role of generation of structural/functional proteins in correlation with its IRES. In fact, the gag polyprotein encoded by the Gag IRES associates with 5′ UTR of HIV mRNA, forming a gRNA–Gag complex that inhibits ribosomal scanning, decreases translation and increases encapsidation (Chamond, et al., 2010). The ability to switch from cap-dependent to IRES-dependent translation by HIV is most closely related to that of cellular IRES-containing mRNA, which will be addressed in the next section.

3.7. IRES of Cellular mRNA

While many of the viral IRES-containing mRNAs have been studied quite extensively, much less is known about cellular IRES-containing mRNA. It's estimated that ~10-15% of cellular mRNA possesses the ability to translate via cap-independent mechanisms (Graber, et al., 2009, Johannes, et al., 1999, Qin & Sarnow, 2004). The cellular genes that contain IRESs in their mRNAs generally have been shown to code for proteins that are involved in growth, proliferation, apoptosis, stress response, differentiation and cell cycle regulation (Komar & Hatzoglou, 2011). Cellular IRESs often are found in mRNA containing long 5′UTRs that are rich in GC and have complex secondary structures (Holcik, et al., 2005). Often, in the mRNA structure there are also multiple short modules whose combined effects are IRES activation, as well as pseudoknots, that are believed to be inhibitory in function (Stoneley & Willis, 2004). However, to date there is no consensus structural or conformational motifs that are conserved among cellular IRES that would make them easily identifiable. Unlike their structurally stable viral counterparts, cellular IRESs identified to date follow a pattern of less structure corresponding to enhanced IRES activation (Filbin & Kieft, 2009). Like their viral counterparts, cellular IRESs are able to initiate translation without many of the canonical translational factors, particularly cap-binding factors such as eIF4E (Hellen & Sarnow, 2001). Cellular IRESs also utilize ITAFs to replace canonical translational factors rendered unavailable. Many of the ITAFs utilized by the cell are also utilized by viruses, including PTB, UNR, poly-(rC)-binding protein 1 (PCBP1), La autoantigen and hnRNPC1/C2, many of which shuttle between the nucleus and cytoplasm (Stoneley & Willis, 2004). Dicistronic cellular mRNA containing IRESs were inactive when introduced directly into the cytoplasm, suggesting the possibility of prerequisite nuclear ITAF-IRES complex formation for IRES activation, at least for apoptotic genes (Spriggs, et al., 2005). Interestingly, much like the highly evolved HIV IRES, the G2/M phase of the cell cycle (where cap-dependent protein synthesis is inhibited) is important for cell cycle regulatory gene's IRES activation as well, including $p58^{PITSLRE}$ (Stoneley & Willis, 2004).

The notion of cellular mRNAs containing IRESs is not without controversy. The viral shut down of host canonical translation machinery results in an overall reduction in global protein synthesis. However, many host cellular stress responsive mRNAs are still actively translated. This led to the hypothesis that certain select cellular mRNAs contain IRESs in their 5'UTRs. Indeed, there are several cellular mRNAs containing IRESs in their 5'UTR (Gilbert, W.V., 2010). The previous methods used to determine the existence of cellular IRESs have been under some scrutiny as to their capability of truly detecting and confirming actual IRES structures within cellular 5'UTRs. Bicistronic reporter assays where the 5'UTR of the suspected mRNA containing IRES was cloned between two reporter genes are subject to false positives via cryptic promoter artifacts (Gilbert, W.V., 2010). Therefore, future work needs to be done to verify if some cellular genes truly contain IRESs in the 5'UTR of their mRNA.

3.8. DNA virus IRES

Much less studied are the DNA viruses, which transcribe mRNA containing an IRES that translates certain proteins independent of the cap structure, much like their cellular IRES counterparts. To date, there are six known DNA viruses known to contain IRESs, four of which belong to the *Herpesviridae* family (http://iresite.org/), particularily the latent gammaherpesviruses (Coleman, et al., 2003). The most well documented DNA viral IRES is that of the Kaposi's sarcoma herpes virus (KSHV) (fig.2) (Bieleski, and Talbot, 2001) while others include Herpes simplex virus (Griffiths, A. and Coen, D. M., 2005) and Marek's disease virus (Tahiri-Alaoui, et al., 2009) to name a few. The KSHV IRES is representative of most IRESs in the *Herpesviridae* family in that it is similar in structure to that of HCV, containing two major stem loops (Beales, et al., 2003). Although most IRESs identified are located in the 5'UTR, the KSHV IRES is found in the coding sequence of the upstream cistron, vCyclin (Bieleski & Talbot, 2001). Interestingly, the KSHV IRES is translational active during viral latency and codes for a viral FLICE (FADD [Fas-associated death domain]-like interleukin-1 beta-converting enzyme)-inhibitory protein, vFLIP (Flice inhibitory protein homolog), which inhibits caspase activation and also promotes proliferation (Bieleski & Talbot, 2001). Again, the trend for IRES involved in cell growth/proliferation is consistent in DNA viruses as well. While there remains quite a bit yet to be discovered in our understanding of the structure and function of IRES elements in translation initiation, clearly, the stress-induced shift from cap-dependent to IRES-dependent translation is a vital strategy for the cell and virus to survive unfavorable conditions.

*For a comprehensive review of current known IRESs, the reader may refer to http://iresite.org/.

4. Mechanisms of survival: Switching translation initiation from cap-dependent to IRES-dependent

As discussed above, both cells and viruses utilize a strategy for survival by switching translation initiation from cap-dependent to IRES-dependent. During this process, both the canonical translation factors and ITAFs utilized by a given virus are dependent upon IRES structure, as it is highly indicative of function. For example, structural components found in the mRNA of Hepatitus C virus (HCV) IRES are able to mimic the function of certain canonical translational factors. (Sonenberg, et al., 2009). HCV also utilizes litagin and the oncogenes MCT-1/DENR as ITAFs, supplementing the function canonical factors of eIF1, eIF1A, eIF3 and eIF3 (Skabkin, et al., 2010). Picornaviruses and others have demonstrated the capability of influencing the cell and manipulating its translational components, favoring its own translation and replication. Viral translation includes modulating not only canonical eukaryotic initiation factors, but also their binding proteins as well. The eukaryotic translation initiation components modulated during infection are specific to a given virus and can vary quite substantially. On the other hand, host cells utilize highly conserved mechanisms of defense to a variety of stimuli, including viral infection, osmotic shock, toxin, heat shock, etc. Here, we summarize some of the recent advances in our knowledge of the mechanisms utilized by viruses and cells to promote IRES-dependent translation allowing survival during unfavorable conditions.

4.1. Cleavage of translation initiation factors by viral proteases

In order to influence cellular translation, viral proteases often target the cellular canonical translation initiation factors for cleavage. The early identified such factor is eIF4G (later called eIF4GI), which along with eIF4E, constitute critical translational factors targeted during several viral infections. This is evident by the highly specific cleavage of eIF4GI during picornaviral infection, which generates a truncated C-terminal form that is unable to bind eIF4E (Svitkin, et al., 2005). Another translation initiation factor eIF4GII as well as the polyA binding protein (PABP), a protein facilitating the formation of a closed translation initiation loop by interaction of the 5′ and 3′ ends of the mRNA, has been reported to be cleaved by picornaviral 2A (Gradi, et al., 1998, Joachims, et al., 1999). All these cleavages often correspond with a translational shift to IRES-dependent translation (Redondo, et al., 2011 Welnowska, et al., 2011), rendering the eIFs incapable of performing cap-dependent translation. Another group also showed that the shift in translation seen during the later phase of poliovirus infection is not entirely due to phosphorylation (inactivation) of eIF2α (see discussion in later session), but may also depend upon protease 3C activation and cleavage of another translation initiation factor, eIF5B, to a C-terminal truncated version thought to replace eIF2 during translation (White, et al., 2011). In all these cleavage events, viral protein synthesis was increased during periods of global protein suppression caused by eIF2α phosphorylation, however the mechanism may likely be a combination of both 2A and 3C proteolytic activity. The apparent shift in translation occurs at times during infection when viral proteases are highly expressed. These observations are representative of viral evolution in correspondence to cellular anti-viral mechanisms. Other factors such as FMDV protease 3C mediated specific cleavage of eIF4AI but not eIF4AII highlight the target specificity that has quite often evolved to be viral specific (Li, et al., 2001).

4.2. Cleavage of translation initiation factors by caspases

Like their viral counterparts, the cell utilizes a subset of proteases, the caspases, to cleave some translation initiation factors. The activation of the caspases often corresponds to the induction of apoptosis (Cohen, 1997). It has been demonstrated in cells committed to apoptosis that caspases cleave eIF4E-BP1, which enhances its capability to bind and inhibit eIF4E, thereby inhibiting cap-dependent translation (Tee & Proud, 2002). eIF2 is cleaved at its α subunit by caspase-3, further implicating its critical role in translational control (Satoh, et al., 1999). Caspase-3 was also shown to cleave scaffolding protein eIF4GI, inhibiting its eIF4E binding capabilities, as well as cleaving its homolog DAP5 (death associated protein 5, also called NAT1/p97), both during conditions of apoptosis (Henis-Korenblit, et al., 2000, Marissen, et al., 1998). Perhaps not surprisingly, viral strategies target many of the same canonical translation initiation factors (including all of those mentioned here) and is reflective of similar strategies used by the cell defense system, marking a translational switch to cap-independent translation during stress and promoting translation of apoptotic inducing genes.

4.3. Phosphorylation of eukaryotic initiation factors and co-factors

The cell has multiple signaling mechanisms that it utilizes to influence translation. Phosphorylation is perhaps the one of most common and conserved method utilized by the cell. Protein kinases involved in cellular stress response regulation such as PKR, PERK, GCN2, and HRT (heme-regulated kinases) all conservatively deactivate eIF2 on its α subunit in response to their respective stress stimulus, influencing the shift to cap-independent translation (Sonenberg, et al., 2009). This multi-faceted capability of the cell to redundantly suppress cap-dependent translation initiation through phosphorylation of eIF2α is quite intriguing and spans multiple disease and stress conditions. This highlights the critical importance of translation initiation in cell fate and physiology. eIF4E also is a highly targeted translation factor during viral infection as well as during other conditions of stress, such as heat shock, ER stress, oxidative stress, etc. In fact, eIF4E and its regulatory protein eIF4E-BP have been utilized as predictive biomarkers in breast cancer (Coleman, et al., 2009). This is because it functions as the cap binding translation initiation factor thought to be the rate-limiting step of translation and therefore is a key component to cap-dependent translation (Gingras, et al., 1999). The availability of eIF4E (which is highly cytoplasmic) to participate in cap-dependent translation is regulated by several factors, the most apparent being 4E-BP, which binds eIF4E and is involved in its localization to the nucleus and in stress granules, rendering it inactive (Sukarieh, et al., 2009). 4E-BP is regulated by phosphorylation by the highly conserved serine/threonine kinase (mammalian target of rapamycin (mTOR)), which decreases its affinity to eIF4E (Kimball & Jefferson, 2004), thus resulting in increased levels of protein translated cap-dependently due to increased availability of cap binding protein eIF4E. However, hypophosphorylated 4E-BPs binds strongly to eIF4E and thus attenuates cap-dependent translation. Similarly, eIF4G has been shown to be phosphorylated by protein kinase C (PKCα) through the Ras-ERK pathway, resulting in increase affinity for eIF4E binding and enhanced eIF4E-mnk1 modulating capabilities (Dobrikov, et al., 2011). Therefore, phosphorylation modulated by stress stimulus (i.e. heat shock, osmotic stress, ER stress, viral infection) results in stress pathway activation (ERK, MAPK, PKR, etc.) and subsequent phosphorylation of a translation initiation component (i.e. eIF4E, eIF4G, eIF2, 4E-BP) which represses or enhances its function and contributes to the translational switch between IRES and cap-dependent modes.

4.4. eIF4E-binding Proteins and other associated proteins compete with eIF4E to inhibit cap-dependent translation

Another similar mechanism for controlling the shift of translation initiation is the up-regulation of 4E-BP production, which affects the mRNA 5′-cap recognition process of eIF4F. In cap-dependent translation, eIF4E forms the eIF4F complex along with translation initiation factors eIF4A, eIF4B and eIF4G (Merrick, 1992). The interaction between eIF4G and eIF4E in the eIF4F complex is inhibited by 4E-BPs (also called eIF4E homolog). Recently, it was reported that Argonaut (Ago) protein, a core component of RISC, binds directly to the cap structure and that this binding competes with eIF4E and results in inhibition of cap-dependent translation initiation (Kiriakidou, et al., 2007). The central domain of Ago exhibits limited sequence homology to the eIF4E and contains two aromatic residues that could function in a similar manner to those in eIF4E in interaction with the cap structure. However, this conclusion has been questioned by another study (Eulalio, et al., 2008). Another factor eIF6 has been reported to associate with Ago protein and the large ribosomal subunits (Chendrimada, et al., 2007). By binding to the large ribosomal subunit, eIF6 prevents this subunit from prematurely joining with the small ribosomal subunit. Thus, if Ago2 recruits eIF6, then the large and small ribosomal subunits might not be able to associate, causing translation to be repressed (Chendrimada, et al., 2007). Drosophila Cup also suppresses cap dependent translation by binding eIF4E at the same conserved sequence utilized by 4E-BPs (Nakamura, et al., 2004).

4.5. The Role of microRNAs (miRNA) in translational control

Many viruses also indirectly influence the availability of cellular translational components. miRNAs are small (~20-24 nts) non-coding RNAs that bind partially complimentary mRNA sequences (mostly in the 3′UTR and less so in the 5′UTR and coding regions) resulting in translational repression and mRNA degradation or (in instances of cellular quiescence) translational activation (Fabian, et al., Sonenberg, et al., 2009). They are loaded onto target mRNA sequences by an RNA induced silencing complex (RISC), whose major component proteins are the Ago protein family (Sonenberg, et al., 2009). It was recently shown that Ago proteins are required for miR-122 activated translation during HCV infection (Roberts, et al., 2011). In addition, as mention earlier, Ago binds competitively to the cap structure of mRNA to inhibit cap-dependent initiation of translation. It is not surprising that miRNA mediated repression has been shown to be specific to a given mRNA containing both a cap structure and poly-(A) tail, in fact mRNA without a cap structure or poly-(A) tail were resistant to miRNA-mediated repression (Humphreys, et al., 2005). miRNA modulated repression takes place in processing (P)-bodies that contain decapping enzymes (see discussion in a later section), further supporting the role of miRNA in suppressing cap-dependent translation initiation (Sonenberg, et al., 2009). Viruses have been shown to influence the expression of select miRNAs (Ho, et al., 2011, Humphreys, et al., 2005, Lei, et al., 2010), which are often involved in the inhibition of cap-dependent translation (Humphreys, et al., 2005, Walters, et al., 2009) lending to a virally influenced shift to IRES-mediated translation. In the early study of the mechanism of translation suppression using an artificial miRNA targeting CXCR4, the cap/4E-BP and the poly-(A) tail of mRNA were all found to play an important role because they are each necessary but not sufficient for full miRNA-mediated repression of translation. Replacing the cap with a viral IRES impairs miRNA-mediated suppression. These results suggest that miRNAs interfere with the initiation step of translation and implicate 4E-BP as a molecular target (Humphreys, et al., 2005). This finding was further solidified by a recent study, which demonstrated that enterovirus 71 (EV71) infection up-regulated miR-141 expression and resulted in a shift from cap-dependent to cap-independent translation initiation by targeting 4E-BP. As EV71 RNA translates through a cap-independent, IRES mechanism, this targeting enhanced EV71 replication (Ho, et al., 2011). Another miRNA, miR-2, has also been reported to utilize a similar mechanism to target the cap structure (Zdanowicz, et al., 2009). This study screened a library of chemical m^7GpppN cap structures and identified defined modifications of the triphosphate backbone that augment miRNA-mediated inhibition of translation but are "neutral" toward to general cap-dependent translation. Interestingly, these caps also augment inhibition by 4E-BP, suggesting that miR-2's cap targeting is through a mechanism related to the 4E-BP class of translation regulators (Zdanowicz, et al., 2009).

The above studies clearly support the notion of a virally influenced translational shift favoring cap-independent translation. This is achieved through several mechanisms including indirectly, such as up-regulating the expression of certain miRNAs that repress cap-binding canonical translation initiation factors in the eI4F complex (Mathonnet, et al., 2007). Here, it is worth mentioning that viruses with a nuclear DNA phase, including HIV and Herpesviruses, may generate virally derived miRNAs during the infection cycle (Griffiths-Jones, et al., 2008, Pilakka-Kanthikeel, et al., 2011), however, whether HIV generates miRNAs is still contentious as other labs have not been able to verify them experimentally (Lin., Cullen, 2007, Pfeffer, et al., 2005). Intriguingly, the cytoplasmic RNA tick-borne encephalitis virus (TBEV), a member of the *Flaviviridae* family, has been shown to encode its own viral miRNA when a heterologous miRNA-precursor stem-loop was artificially introduced into the RNA viral genome (Rouha, et al., 2010). This opens up the possibility of other cytoplasmic RNA viruses to have similar capabilities. It may be possible to artificially introduce miRNAs into viral genomes, which may in turn be able to shut down viral replication by targeting mRNAs of specific translation initiation factors required by the virus, which generate a new avenue for generating vaccines and attenuating viral replication. Clearly miRNAs represent an exciting and newly emerging dimension to our study and understanding of viruses and their ability to manipulate cellular translation during infection and other conditions of stress.

4.6. Activation of decapping enzymes

Decapping of mRNA by decapping enzymes represents another modality by which cap-dependent translation is suppressed by the cell. To date, two decapping enzymes have been identified: Dcp2 which cleaves mRNA at the cap site and the scavenger decapping enzyme (DcpS) that hydrolyzes the cap structure, both function to facilitate the subsequent degradation of target cap-dependent mRNA (Li & Kiledjian, 2011). Enzymatic decapping of select mRNAs is influenced by miRNA. As mentioned above, miRNA mediated repression occurs in P-bodies where Ago proteins have been shown to co-immunoprecipitate with decapping enzymes, suggesting their close association (Parker & Sheth, 2007). P bodies also contain other proteins including, GW182, the CAF1-CCR4-NOT deadenylase complex, the decapping activators (e.g., DCP1, EDC3, Ge-1), and the RNA helicase RCK/p54, all of which have been implicated in miRNA function (Eulalio, et al., 2007, Parker, et al., 2007). Decapping enzymes functions may also be modulated by cell signaling pathways and are also found in stress granules. Indeed, the phosphorylation of the decapping enzyme DCP2 has been shown to influence stress granule formation and its availability in P-bodies (Yoon, et al., 2010). HCV has been shown to selectively disrupt P-body components during infection leaving the decapping enzyme DCP2, active and functioning to highjack other translational machinery for the enhancement of its own translation (Ariumi, et al., 2011). Therefore, not surprisingly, viruses modulate decapping enzyme activity to favor their translation.

5. Conclusions and perspectives

It is evident that more and more newly discovered cellular mRNAs contain IRESs and can participate in a shift in translation from global, cap-dependent to IRES-driven initiation during ER stress. One of the most well studied causes of ER stress is viral infection, which can globally shut down cap-dependent translation initiation by different mechanisms. To adapt to unfavorable stress conditions, both cell and virus (e.g., HIV) need to adjust their mode of translation initiation by switching from the cap-dependent to cap-independent mechanism. As picornaviruses do not have a cap structure, its RNA translation will not be inhibited; instead it will be enhanced because more translational machinery is available due to the shutoff of global cap-dependent translation, achieved by a number of mechanisms.

During transient ER stress, the IRES-containing cellular mRNAs that are responsible for cell survival/growth, such as BiP and Bcl-2, will be selectively translated by an IRES-dependent mechanism, utilizing ITAFs in place of inhibited canonical translational factors. This mechanism allows cells to respond rapidly to the transient changes in growth conditions and to delay apoptosis. Once the stress is removed, cellular homeostasis is restored. However, during prolonged or severe stress, such as in persistent infection of picornaviruses, the pro-death genes, such as Apaf1, DAP5, CHOP, p53, etc., are also selectively translated by the same IRES-driven mechanism, allowing the cells to fine-tune their responses to cellular stress and, if conditions for cell survival are not restored, to proceed with final execution of apoptosis (Fig. 2).

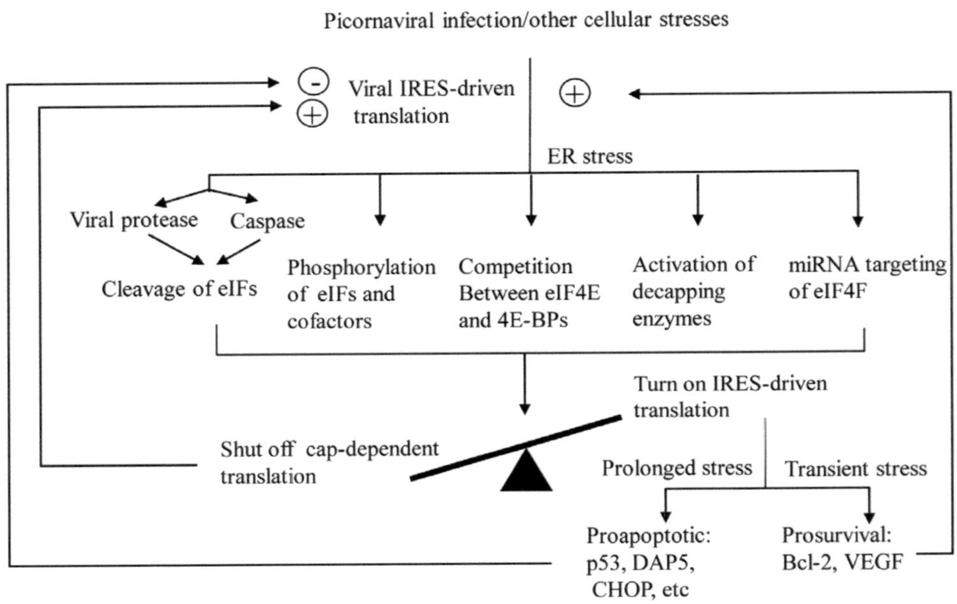

Figure 2. The proposed model for the switch of translation initiation from cap-dependent to IRES-dependent during picornaviral infection or other cellular stresses. Positive and negative feedback loops are indicated by plus and minus signs, respectively.

Although some mechanisms on the switch of the translation initiation and subsequent selective translation have been described, many questions are still unanswered: for example, what are the regulators for selecting the pro-survival or proapoptotic genes? In other words, do these genes contain different binding sequences for their specific regulators? Previous studies using a polysome system predicted that approximately 10-15% of the cellular mRNAs contain IRESs (Carter, 2000, Graber, et al., Qin, et al., 2004); thus, more IRES-containing cellular mRNAs will need to be discovered to fully understand the underlying mechanisms of IRES-dependent translational control. In the shutoff of global cap-dependent translation, cleavages of cellular proteins are known to play an important role. In this regard, besides the viral proteases and the activated cellular caspases, other cellular proteases responsible for the cleavage of translation initiation factors need to be identified.

In addition, efforts to discover other cellular target proteins that are specifically cleaved during cellular stress are another future area of research. Identification of these target proteins may uncover the linkage between translational control and pathogenesis. Recently, miRNAs, as a group of new regulators of gene expression, were found to be involved in regulation of the shift of translation initiation. However, the research in this direction is just emerging. More studies on the interactions between miRNAs and their target mRNAs encoding translation initiation factors need to be carried out. Indeed, the biological implications of the selective translation of specific genes are clearly important. Since the IRES-mediated translation initiation links with many pathophysiological conditions, such as hypoxia, heat shock, toxin, metabolic disorder, viral infection, etc., the failure of maintaining the balance between the cap-dependent and cap-independent translation initiation may cause human diseases, such as heart disease, stroke, diabetes, and viral induced diseases. Similarly, dysregulated apoptosis has been associated with many human disorders, ranging from autoimmune diseases, neurodegeneration to a variety of cancers. Therefore, better understanding how the translational control determines the cellular response to stress will provide novel insights into the molecular pathogenesis of human disorders and will likely eventually lead to the development of effective therapeutics.

Author details

Paul J Hanson, Huifang M. Zhang, Maged Gomaa Hemida, Xin Ye, Ye Qiu
and Decheng Yang
Department of Pathology and Laboratory Medicine, University of British Columbia, The Institute for Heart and Lung Health, St. Paul's Hospital, Vancouver, Canada

Acknowledgement

This work was supported by grants from the Canadian Institutes of Health Research and the Heart and Stroke Foundation of BC and Yukon. Dr. Maged Gomaa Hemida is a recipient of the CIHR-IMPACT postdoctoral training fellowship and the Heart and Stroke foundation of Canada postdoctoral training fellowship. Xin Ye is supported by a UGF Award from the University of British Columbia.

6. References

Ahmed, R. and Duncan, R. F.I (2004). Translational regulation of Hsp90 mRNA. AUG-proximal 5'-untranslated region elements essential for preferential heat shock translation. *J Biol Chem*, 279,48I 49919-30.

Ali, I. K., McKendrick, L., Morley, S. J. and Jackson, R. J.I (2001). Activity of the hepatitis A virus *IRES* requires association between the cap-binding translation initiation factor (eIF4E) and eIF4G. *J Virol*, 75,17I 7854-63.

Ariumi, Y., Kuroki, M., Kushima, Y., Osugi, K., Hijikata, M., Maki, M., Ikeda, M. and Kato, N.I (2011). Hepatitis C virus hijacks P-body and stress granule components around lipid droplets. *J Virol*, 85,14I 6882-92.

Belsham, G. J.I (2009). Divergent picornavirus IRES elements. *Virus Res*, 139,2I 183-92.

Bieleski, L. and Talbot, S.J. (2001). Kaposi's sarcoma-associated herpesvirus vCyclin open reading frame contains an internal ribosome entry J Virol. 75 (4):1864-9

Bollo, M., Paredes, R. M., Holstein, D., Zheleznova, N., Camacho, P. and Lechleiter, J. D.I (2010). Calcineurin interacts with PERK and dephosphorylates calnexin to relieve ER stress in mammals and frogs. *PLoS One*, 5,8I e11925.

Burikhanov, R., Zhao, Y., Goswami, A., Qiu, S., Schwarze, S. R. and Rangnekar, V. M.I (2009). The tumor suppressor Par-4 activates an extrinsic pathway for apoptosis. *Cell*, 138,2I 377-88.

Carter, M., Kuhn, K., and Sarnow, P. (2000). Translational Control of Gene Expression. Cold Spring Harbor Laboratory Press, New York

Chakrabarti, A., Chen, A. W. and Varner, J. D.I (2011). A review of the mammalian unfolded protein response. *Biotechnol Bioeng*.

Chau, D. H., Yuan, J., Zhang, H., Cheung, P., Lim, T., Liu, Z., Sall, A. and Yang, D.I (2007). Coxsackievirus B3 proteases 2A and 3C induce apoptotic cell death through mitochondrial injury and cleavage of eIF4GI but not DAP5/p97/NAT1. *Apoptosis*, 12,3I 513-24.

Chendrimada, T. P., Finn, K. J., Ji, X., Baillat, D., Gregory, R. I., Liebhaber, S. A., Pasquinelli, A. E. and Shiekhattar, R.I (2007). MicroRNA silencing through RISC recruitment of eIF6. *Nature*, 447,7146I 823-8.

Cohen, G. M.I (1997). Caspases: the executioners of apoptosis. *Biochem J*, 326 (Pt 1)1-16.

Coleman, L. J., Peter, M. B., Teall, T. J., Brannan, R. A., Hanby, A. M., Honarpisheh, H., Shaaban, A. M., Smith, L., Speirs, V., Verghese, E. T., McElwaine, J. N. and Hughes, T. A.I (2009).Combined analysis of eIF4E and 4E-binding protein expression predicts breast cancer survival and estimates eIF4E activity. *Br J Cancer*, 100,9I 1393-9.

de Breyne, S., Yu, Y., Pestova, T. V. and Hellen, C. U.I (2008). Factor requirements for translation initiation on the Simian picornavirus internal ribosomal entry site. *RNA*, 14,2I 367-80.

Dobrikov, M., Dobrikova, E., Shveygert, M. and Gromeier, M.I (2011). Phosphorylation of eukaryotic translation initiation factor 4G1 (eIF4G1) by protein kinase C{alpha} regulates eIF4G1 binding to Mnk1. *Mol Cell Biol*, 31,14I 2947-59.

Ekchariyawat, P., Thitithanyanont, A., Sirisinha, S. and Utaisincharoen, P.I (2011). Apoptosis induced by avian H5N1 virus in human monocyte-derived macrophages involves TRAIL-inducing caspase-10 activation. *Innate Immun*.

Etchison, D., Milburn, S. C., Edery, I., Sonenberg, N. and Hershey, J. W.I (1982). Inhibition of HeLa cell protein synthesis following poliovirus infection correlates with the proteolysis of a 220,000-dalton polypeptide associated with eucaryotic initiation factor 3 and a cap binding protein complex. *J Biol Chem*, 257,24I 14806-10.

Eulalio, A., Behm-Ansmant, I. and Izaurralde, E.I (2007). P bodies: at the crossroads of post-transcriptional pathways. *Nat Rev Mol Cell Biol*, 8,1I 9-22.

Eulalio, A., Huntzinger, E. and Izaurralde, E.I (2008). GW182 interaction with Argonaute is essential for miRNA-mediated translational repression and mRNA decay. *Nat Struct Mol Biol*, 15,4I 346-53.

Fabian, M. R., Sonenberg, N. and Filipowicz, W.I (2010). Regulation of mRNA translation and stability by microRNAs. *Annu Rev Biochem*, 79351-79.

Fels, D. R. and Koumenis, C.I (2006). The PERK/eIF2alpha/ATF4 module of the UPR in hypoxia resistance and tumor growth. *Cancer Biol Ther*, 5,7I 723-8.

Fernandez-Miragall, O., Lopez de Quinto, S. and Martinez-Salas, E.I (2009). Relevance of RNA structure for the activity of picornavirus IRES elements. *Virus Res*, 139,2I 172-82.

Filbin, M. E. and Kieft, J. S.I (2009). Toward a structural understanding of IRES RNA function. *Curr Opin Struct Biol*, 19,3I 267-76.

Gilbert, W.V. (2010). Alternative ways to think about cellular internal ribosome entry. *Journal of Biological Chemistry*. 285, 38, 29033-38.

Gingras, A. C., Raught, B. and Sonenberg, N.I (1999). eIF4 initiation factors: effectors of mRNA recruitment to ribosomes and regulators of translation. *Annu Rev Biochem*, 68913-63.

Gotoh, T., Terada, K., Oyadomari, S. and Mori, M.I (2004). hsp70-DnaJ chaperone pair prevents nitric oxide- and CHOP-induced apoptosis by inhibiting translocation of Bax to mitochondria. *Cell Death Differ*, 11,4I 390-402.

Graber, T. E., Baird, S. D., Kao, P. N., Mathews, M. B. and Holcik, M.I (2009). NF45 functions as an IRES trans-acting factor that is required for translation of cIAP1 during the unfolded protein response. *Cell Death Differ*, 17,4I 719-29.

Gradi, A., Svitkin, Y. V., Imataka, H. and Sonenberg, N.I (1998). Proteolysis of human eukaryotic translation initiation factor eIF4GII, but not eIF4GI, coincides with the shutoff of host protein synthesis after poliovirus infection. *Proc Natl Acad Sci U S A*, 95,19I 11089-94.

Griffiths-Jones, S., Saini, H. K., van Dongen, S. and Enright, A. J.I (2008). miRBase: tools for microRNA genomics. *Nucleic Acids Res*, 36,Database issueI D154-8.

Harding, H. P., Calfon, M., Urano, F., Novoa, I. and Ron, D.I (2002). Transcriptional and translational control in the Mammalian unfolded protein response. *Annu Rev Cell Dev Biol*, 18575-99.

Hart, L. S. and El-Deiry, W. S.I (2009). Cell death: a new Par-4 the TRAIL. *Cell*, 138,2I 220-2.

Hellen, C. U. and Sarnow, P.I (2001). Internal ribosome entry sites in eukaryotic mRNA molecules. *Genes Dev*, 15,13I 1593-612.

Hellen, C. U.I (2009). IRES-induced conformational changes in the ribosome and the mechanism of translation initiation by internal ribosomal entry. *Biochim Biophys Acta*, 1789,9-10I 558-70.

Henis-Korenblit, S., Strumpf, N. L., Goldstaub, D. and Kimchi, A.I (2000). A novel form of DAP5 protein accumulates in apoptotic cells as a result of caspase cleavage and internal ribosome entry site-mediated translation. *Mol Cell Biol*, 20,2I 496-506.

Henis-Korenblit, S., Shani, G., Sines, T., Marash, L., Shohat, G. and Kimchi, A.I (2002). The caspase-cleaved DAP5 protein supports internal ribosome entry site-mediated translation of death proteins. *Proc Natl Acad Sci U S A*, 99,8I 5400-5.

Hernandez, G., Vazquez-Pianzola, P., Sierra, J. M. and Rivera-Pomar, R.I (2004). Internal ribosome entry site drives cap-independent translation of reaper and heat shock protein 70 mRNAs in Drosophila embryos. *RNA*, 10,11I 1783-97.

Hetz, C., Bernasconi, P., Fisher, J., Lee, A. H., Bassik, M. C., Antonsson, B., Brandt, G. S., Iwakoshi, N. N., Schinzel, A., Glimcher, L. H. and Korsmeyer, S. J.I (2006). Proapoptotic BAX and BAK modulate the unfolded protein response by a direct interaction with IRE1alpha. *Science*, 312,5773I 572-6.

Ho, B. C., Yu, S. L., Chen, J. J., Chang, S. Y., Yan, B. S., Hong, Q. S., Singh, S., Kao, C. L., Chen, H. Y., Su, K. Y., Li, K. C., Cheng, C. L., Cheng, H. W., Lee, J. Y., Lee, C. N. and Yang, P. C.I (2011). Enterovirus-induced miR-141 contributes to shutoff of host protein translation by targeting the translation initiation factor eIF4E. *Cell Host Microbe*, 9,1I 58-69.

Holcik, M. and Sonenberg, N.I (2005). Translational control in stress and apoptosis. *Nat Rev Mol Cell Biol*, 6,4I 318-27.

Hollien, J., Lin, J. H., Li, H., Stevens, N., Walter, P. and Weissman, J. S.I (2009). Regulated Ire1-dependent decay of messenger RNAs in mammalian cells. *J Cell Biol*, 186,3I 323-31.

Humphreys, D. T., Westman, B. J., Martin, D. I. and Preiss, T.I (2005). MicroRNAs control translation initiation by inhibiting eukaryotic initiation factor 4E/cap and poly (A) tail function. *Proc Natl Acad Sci U S A*, 102,47I 16961-6.

Jackson, R. J., Hellen, C. U. and Pestova, T. V.I (2010). The mechanism of eukaryotic translation initiation and principles of its regulation. *Nat Rev Mol Cell Biol*, 11,2I 113-27.

Jang, C. J., Lo, M. C. and Jan, E.I (2009). Conserved element of the dicistrovirus IGR IRES that mimics an E-site tRNA/ribosome interaction mediates multiple functions. *J Mol Biol*, 387,1I 42-58.

Jang, S. K., Krausslich, H. G., Nicklin, M. J., Duke, G. M., Palmenberg, A. C. and Wimmer, E.I (1988). A segment of the 5' nontranslated region of encephalomyocarditis virus RNA directs internal entry of ribosomes during in vitro translation. *J Virol*, 62,8I 2636-43.

Jang, S. K., Pestova, T. V., Hellen, C. U., Witherell, G. W. and Wimmer, E.I (1990). Cap-independent translation of picornavirus RNAs: structure and function of the internal ribosomal entry site. *Enzyme*, 44,1-4I 292-309.

Jang, S. K.I (2006). Internal initiation: IRES elements of picornaviruses and hepatitis c virus. *Virus Res*, 119,1I 2-15.

Joachims, M., Van Breugel, P. C. and Lloyd, R. E.I (1999). Cleavage of poly (A)-binding protein by enterovirus proteases concurrent with inhibition of translation in vitro. *J Virol*, 73,1I 718-27.

Johannes, G., Carter, M. S., Eisen, M. B., Brown, P. O. and Sarnow, P.I (1999). Identification of eukaryotic mRNAs that are translated at reduced cap binding complex eIF4F concentrations using a cDNA microarray. *Proc Natl Acad Sci U S A*, 96,23I 13118-23.

John, L., Thomas, S., Herchenroder, O., Putzer, B. M. and Schaefer, S.I (2011). Hepatitis E virus ORF2 protein activates the pro-apoptotic gene CHOP and anti-apoptotic heat shock proteins. *PLoS One*, 6,9I e25378.

Kimball, S. R. and Jefferson, L. S.I (2004). Regulation of global and specific mRNA translation by oral administration of branched-chain amino acids. *Biochem Biophys Res Commun*, 313,2I 423-7.

Kiriakidou, M., Tan, G. S., Lamprinaki, S., De Planell-Saguer, M., Nelson, P. T. and Mourelatos, Z.I (2007). An mRNA m7G cap binding-like motif within human Ago2 represses translation. *Cell*, 129,6I 1141-51.

Komar, A. A. and Hatzoglou, M.I (2005). Internal ribosome entry sites in cellular mRNAs: mystery of their existence. *J Biol Chem*, 280,25I 23425-8.

Komar, A. A. and Hatzoglou, M.I (2011). Cellular IRES-mediated translation: the war of ITAFs in pathophysiological states. *Cell Cycle*, 10,2I 229-40.

Labadie, K., Pelletier, I., Saulnier, A., Martin, J. and Colbere-Garapin, F.I (2004). Poliovirus mutants excreted by a chronically infected hypogammaglobulinemic patient establish persistent infections in human intestinal cells. *Virology*, 318,1I 66-78.

Lamphear, B. J., Yan, R., Yang, F., Waters, D., Liebig, H. D., Klump, H., Kuechler, E., Skern, T. and Rhoads, R. E.I (1993). Mapping the cleavage site in protein synthesis initiation factor eIF-4 gamma of the 2A proteases from human Coxsackievirus and rhinovirus. *J Biol Chem*, 268,26I 19200-3.

Lee, A. H., Iwakoshi, N. N. and Glimcher, L. H.I (2003). XBP-1 regulates a subset of endoplasmic reticulum resident chaperone genes in the unfolded protein response. *Mol Cell Biol*, 23,21I 7448-59.

Lee, K., Tirasophon, W., Shen, X., Michalak, M., Prywes, R., Okada, T., Yoshida, H., Mori, K. and Kaufman, R. J.I (2002). IRE1-mediated unconventional mRNA splicing and S2P-mediated ATF6 cleavage merge to regulate XBP1 in signaling the unfolded protein response. *Genes Dev*, 16,4I 452-66.

Lei, X., Bai, Z., Ye, F., Huang, Y. and Gao, S. J.I (2010). Regulation of herpesvirus lifecycle by viral microRNAs. *Virulence*, 1,5I 433-5.

Lewis, S. M., Cerquozzi, S., Graber, T. E., Ungureanu, N. H., Andrews, M. and Holcik, M.I (2008). The eIF4G homolog DAP5/p97 supports the translation of select mRNAs during endoplasmic reticulum stress. *Nucleic Acids Res*, 36,1I 168-78.

Li, W., Ross-Smith, N., Proud, C. G. and Belsham, G. J.I (2001). Cleavage of translation initiation factor 4AI (eIF4AI) but not eIF4AII by foot-and-mouth disease virus 3C protease: identification of the eIF4AI cleavage site. *FEBS Lett*, 507,1I 1-5.

Li, Y. and Kiledjian, M.I (2011). Regulation of mRNA decapping. *Wiley Interdiscip Rev RNA*, 1,2I 253-65.

Lindeberg, J. and Ebendal, T.I (1999). Use of an internal ribosome entry site for bicistronic expression of Cre recombinase or rtTA transactivator. *Nucleic Acids Res*, 27,6I 1552-4.

Liu, C. Y., Schroder, M. and Kaufman, R. J.I (2000). Ligand-independent dimerization activates the stress response kinases IRE1 and PERK in the lumen of the endoplasmic reticulum. *J Biol Chem*, 275,32I 24881-5.

Locker, N., Chamond, N. and Sargueil, B.I (2010). A conserved structure within the HIV gag open reading frame that controls translation initiation directly recruits the 40S subunit and eIF3. *Nucleic Acids Res*, 39,6I 2367-77.

Ma, Y., Brewer, J. W., Diehl, J. A. and Hendershot, L. M.I (2002). Two distinct stress signaling pathways converge upon the CHOP promoter during the mammalian unfolded protein response. *J Mol Biol*, 318,5I 1351-65.

Malnou, C. E., Werner, A., Borman, A. M., Westhof, E. and Kean, K. M.I (2004). Effects of vaccine strain mutations in domain V of the internal ribosome entry segment compared in the wild type poliovirus type 1 context. *J Biol Chem*, 279,11I 10261-9.

Marcotrigiano, J., Gingras, A. C., Sonenberg, N. and Burley, S. K.I (1999). Cap-dependent translation initiation in eukaryotes is regulated by a molecular mimic of eIF4G. *Mol Cell*, 3,6I 707-16.

Marissen, W. E. and Lloyd, R. E.I (1998). Eukaryotic translation initiation factor 4G is targeted for proteolytic cleavage by caspase 3 during inhibition of translation in apoptotic cells. *Mol Cell Biol*, 18,12I 7565-74.

Mathonnet, G., Fabian, M. R., Svitkin, Y. V., Parsyan, A., Huck, L., Murata, T., Biffo, S., Merrick, W. C., Darzynkiewicz, E., Pillai, R. S., Filipowicz, W., Duchaine, T. F. and Sonenberg, N.I (2007). MicroRNA inhibition of translation initiation in vitro by targeting the cap-binding complex eIF4F. *Science*, 317,5845I 1764-7.

McCullough, K. D., Martindale, J. L., Klotz, L. O., Aw, T. Y. and Holbrook, N. J.I (2001). Gadd153 sensitizes cells to endoplasmic reticulum stress by down-regulating Bcl2 and perturbing the cellular redox state. *Mol Cell Biol*, 21,4I 1249-59.

Mekahli, D., Bultynck, G., Parys, J. B., De Smedt, H. and Missiaen, L.I (2011). Endoplasmic-reticulum calcium depletion and disease. *Cold Spring Harb Perspect Biol*, 3,6I.

Merrick, W. C.I (1992). Mechanism and regulation of eukaryotic protein synthesis. *Microbiol Rev*, 56,2I 291-315.

Morley, S. J., Coldwell, M. J. and Clemens, M. J.I (2005). Initiation factor modifications in the preapoptotic phase. *Cell Death Differ*, 12,6I 571-84.

Nakamura, A., Sato, K. and Hanyu-Nakamura, K.I (2004). Drosophila cup is an eIF4E binding protein that associates with Bruno and regulates oskar mRNA translation in oogenesis. *Dev Cell*, 6,1I 69-78.

Novoa, I., Zeng, H., Harding, H. P. and Ron, D.I (2001). Feedback inhibition of the unfolded protein response by GADD34-mediated dephosphorylation of eIF2alpha. *J Cell Biol*, 153,5I 1011-22.

Ohlmann, T. and Jackson, R. J.I (1999). The properties of chimeric picornavirus IRESes show that discrimination between internal translation initiation sites is influenced by the identity of the IRES and not just the context of the AUG codon. *RNA*, 5,6I 764-78.

Ohlmann, T., Prevot, D., Decimo, D., Roux, F., Garin, J., Morley, S. J. and Darlix, J. L.I (2002). In vitro cleavage of eIF4GI but not eIF4GII by HIV-1 protease and its effects on translation in the rabbit reticulocyte lysate system. *J Mol Biol*, 318,1I 9-20.

Oikawa, D. and Kimata, Y.I (2011). Experimental approaches for elucidation of stress-sensing mechanisms of the IRE1 family proteins. *Methods Enzymol*, 490195-216.

Parker, R. and Sheth, U.I (2007). P bodies and the control of mRNA translation and degradation. *Mol Cell*, 25,5I 635-46.

Pelletier, J. and Sonenberg, N.I (1988). Internal initiation of translation of eukaryotic mRNA directed by a sequence derived from poliovirus RNA. *Nature*, 334,6180I 320-5.

Pestova, T. V., de Breyne, S., Pisarev, A. V., Abaeva, I. S. and Hellen, C. U.I (2008). eIF2-dependent and eIF2-independent modes of initiation on the CSFV IRES: a common role of domain II. *EMBO J*, 27,7I 1060-72.

Pilakka-Kanthikeel, S., Saiyed, Z. M., Napuri, J. and Nair, M. P.I (2011). MicroRNA: implications in HIV, a brief overview. *J Neurovirol*, 17,5I 416-23.

Qin, X. and Sarnow, P.I (2004). Preferential translation of internal ribosome entry site-containing mRNAs during the mitotic cycle in mammalian cells. *J Biol Chem*, 279,14I 13721-8.

Raught, B., Gringas, A.C. (2007). Translational Control in Biology and Medicine Cold Springs Harbor Laboratory Press, New York

Raven, J. F. and Koromilas, A. E.I (2008). PERK and PKR: old kinases learn new tricks. *Cell Cycle*, 7,9I 1146-50.

Redondo, N., Sanz, M. A., Welnowska, E. and Carrasco, L.I (2011). Translation without eIF2 Promoted by Poliovirus 2A Protease. *PLoS One*, 6,10I e25699.

Roberts, A. P., Lewis, A. P. and Jopling, C. L.I (2011). miR-122 activates hepatitis C virus translation by a specialized mechanism requiring particular RNA components. *Nucleic Acids Res*, 39,17I 7716-29.

Rojas-Eisenring, I. A., Cajero-Juarez, M. and del Angel, R. M.I (1995). Cell proteins bind to a linear polypyrimidine-rich sequence within the 5'-untranslated region of rhinovirus 14 RNA. *J Virol*, 69,11I 6819-24.

Rouha, H., Thurner, C. and Mandl, C. W.I (2010). Functional microRNA generated from a cytoplasmic RNA virus. *Nucleic Acids Res*, 38,22I 8328-37.

Satoh, S., Hijikata, M., Handa, H. and Shimotohno, K.I (1999). Caspase-mediated cleavage of eukaryotic translation initiation factor subunit 2alpha. *Biochem J*, 342 (Pt 1)65-70.

Shatsky, I.N., Dmitriev, S. E., Terenin, I. M., Andreev, D. E. (2010). Cap- and IRES-Independent scanning mechanism of translation initiation as an alternative to the concept of cellular IRESs. *Molecules and Cells* 30, 285-293.

Skabkin, M. A., Skabkina, O. V., Dhote, V., Komar, A. A., Hellen, C. U. and Pestova, T. V.I (2010). Activities of Ligatin and MCT-1/DENR in eukaryotic translation initiation and ribosomal recycling. *Genes Dev*, 24,16I 1787-801.

Sonenberg, N. and Hinnebusch, A. G.I (2009). Regulation of translation initiation in eukaryotes: mechanisms and biological targets. *Cell*, 136,4I 731-45.

Spriggs, K. A., Bushell, M., Mitchell, S. A. and Willis, A. E.I (2005). Internal ribosome entry segment-mediated translation during apoptosis: the role of IRES-trans-acting factors. *Cell Death Differ*, 12,6I 585-91.

Stoneley, M. and Willis, A. E.I (2004). Cellular internal ribosome entry segments: structures, trans-acting factors and regulation of gene expression. *Oncogene*, 23,18I 3200-7.

Sukarieh, R., Sonenberg, N. and Pelletier, J.I (2009). The eIF4E-binding proteins are modifiers of cytoplasmic eIF4E relocalization during the heat shock response. *Am J Physiol Cell Physiol*, 296,5I C1207-17.

Svitkin, Y. V., Herdy, B., Costa-Mattioli, M., Gingras, A. C., Raught, B. and Sonenberg, N.I (2005). Eukaryotic translation initiation factor 4E availability controls the switch between cap-dependent and internal ribosomal entry site-mediated translation. *Mol Cell Biol*, 25,23I 10556-65.

Tabas, I. and Ron, D.I (2011). Integrating the mechanisms of apoptosis induced by endoplasmic reticulum stress. *Nat Cell Biol*, 13,3I 184-90.

Tee, A. R. and Proud, C. G.I (2002). Caspase cleavage of initiation factor 4E-binding protein 1 yields a dominant inhibitor of cap-dependent translation and reveals a novel regulatory motif. *Mol Cell Biol*, 22,6I 1674-83.

Vallejos, M., Deforges, J., Plank, T. D., Letelier, A., Ramdohr, P., Abraham, C. G., Valiente-Echeverria, F., Kieft, J. S., Sargueil, B. and Lopez-Lastra, M.I (2011). Activity of the human immunodeficiency virus type 1 cell cycle-dependent internal ribosomal entry site is modulated by IRES trans-acting factors. *Nucleic Acids Res*, 39,14I 6186-200.

Wang, K., Xie, S. and Sun, B.I (2010). Viral proteins function as ion channels. *Biochim Biophys Acta*, 1808,2I 510-5.

Wang, X., Olberding, K. E., White, C. and Li, C.I (2010). Bcl-2 proteins regulate ER membrane permeability to luminal proteins during ER stress-induced apoptosis. *Cell Death Differ*, 18,1I 38-47.

Weill, L., James, L., Ulryck, N., Chamond, N., Herbreteau, C. H., Ohlmann, T. and Sargueil, B.I (2009). A new type of IRES within gag coding region recruits three initiation complexes on HIV-2 genomic RNA. *Nucleic Acids Res*, 38,4I 1367-81.

Welnowska, E., Sanz, M. A., Redondo, N. and Carrasco, L.I (2011). Translation of viral mRNA without active eIF2: the case of picornaviruses. *PLoS One*, 6,7I e22230.

White, J. P., Reineke, L. C. and Lloyd, R. E.I (2011). Poliovirus switches to an eIF2-independent mode of translation during infection. *J Virol*, 85,17I 8884-93.

Yang, D., Wilson, J. E., Anderson, D. R., Bohunek, L., Cordeiro, C., Kandolf, R. and McManus, B. M.I (1997). In vitro mutational and inhibitory analysis of the cis-acting translational elements within the 5' untranslated region of coxsackievirus B3: potential targets for antiviral action of antisense oligomers. *Virology*, 228,1I 63-73.

Yoon, J. H., Choi, E. J. and Parker, R.I (2010). Dcp2 phosphorylation by Ste20 modulates stress granule assembly and mRNA decay in Saccharomyces cerevisiae. *J Cell Biol*, 189,5I 813-27.

Yoshida, H., Okada, T., Haze, K., Yanagi, H., Yura, T., Negishi, M. and Mori, K.I (2001). Endoplasmic reticulum stress-induced formation of transcription factor complex ERSF including NF-Y (CBF) and activating transcription factors 6alpha and 6beta that activates the mammalian unfolded protein response. *Mol Cell Biol*, 21,4I 1239-48.

Zdanowicz, A., Thermann, R., Kowalska, J., Jemielity, J., Duncan, K., Preiss, T., Darzynkiewicz, E. and Hentze, M. W.I (2009). Drosophila miR2 primarily targets the m7GpppN cap structure for translational repression. *Mol Cell*, 35,6I 881-8.

Zhang, H. M., Ye, X., Su, Y., Yuan, J., Liu, Z., Stein, D. A. and Yang, D.I (2010). Coxsackievirus B3 infection activates the unfolded protein response and induces apoptosis through downregulation of p58IPK and activation of CHOP and SREBP1. *J Virol*, 84,17I 8446-59.

Zhu, D. M., Shi, J., Liu, S., Liu, Y. and Zheng, D.I (2011). HIV infection enhances TRAIL-induced cell death in macrophage by down-regulating decoy receptor expression and generation of reactive oxygen species. *PLoS One*, 6,4I e18291.

Chapter 6

Antiviral Replication Agents

Zeinab N. Said and Kouka S. Abdelwahab

Additional information is available at the end of the chapter

http://dx.doi.org/10.5772/53707

1. Introduction

The last few decades have shown a great progress in the development of antiviral agents that were licensed for treatment of Human immunodeficiency virus (HIV), herpesviruses, hepatitis viruses and respiratory viruses. The majority of viral infections clear spontaneously and are not in need for specific medical therapy. However, antiviral chemotherapy is indicated in certain clinical situations including:

Those associated with fatal acute infections: Rabies virus, Respiratory syncytial virus, Hemorrhagic fever viruses (Lassa virus, Yellow fever, Dengue fever, Rift valley fever virus, Ebola virus) and pregnancy viral hepatitis as Hepatitis E virus (HEV) is associated with 20% fatality in pregnant females.

Human viral infections that cause persistent infections (table 1) Human viral infections associated with loss of work hours; Rhinoviruses, Influenza A virus and diarrhoea causing viruses (Calciviruses, Norwalk viruses and Astra viruses).

Family	Virus	Disease or consequence
Retroviridae	Human immunodeficiency virus (HIV)	AIDS
	Human T-cell lymphotrophic virus (HTLV)	Leukaemia
Flaviviridae	Hepatitis C virus (HCV)	Chronic hepatitis, hepatocellular carcinoma
Hepadanaviridae	Hepatitis B virus (HBV)	
Herpesviridae	Herpes simplex virus 1&2 (HSV-1) (HSV-2)	Recurrent mucocutaneous infections, encephalitis
	Varicella zoster virus (VZV)	Recurrent neurological lesions
	Cytomegalovirus (CMV)	Retinitis, pneumonia, encephalitis
	Epstein-Barr virus(EBV)	Lymphoproliferative disorders
Papovaviridae	Human Papillomavirus (HPV)	Cervical carcinoma, warts

Table 1. Common human viruses known to cause persistent infections

2. Targets for antiviral drugs

There are a number of virus-specific processes within the virus replicative cycle or inside a virus infected cell, that have proven to be attractive targets for chemotherapeutic intervention, i.e., virus adsorption and entry into the cells, reverse (RNA to DNA) transcription, viral DNA polymerization, and cellular enzymatic reactions that are associated with viral DNA and RNA synthesis and viral mRNA maturation (i.e., methylation) (De Clercq , 2001). As emphasized by Lorizate and Krausslich, (2011), viruses have to cross the host cell boundary at least twice during their replication, thus alterations of membrane lipid composition can block viral release and entry, and certain lipids act as fusion inhibitors, suggesting a potential as antiviral drugs (Lorizate and Krausslich, 2011).Most DNA viruses replicate in the nucleus and use cellular enzymes, but many DNA viruses have one or more specific viral enzymes for viral DNA replication. These enzymes are potential *targets* for effective antiviral agents. On the other hand, most RNA viruses replicate in the cytoplasm; only positive sense RNA viruses utilize the host machinery exclusively. dsRNA and negative-sense RNA viruses need to encode some, if not all virus specific enzymes for genome replication. while retroviruses have specific reverse transcriptase enzymes. Antiviral agents are effective inhibitors of these virus specific enzymes.

As viruses direct the cell machinery for effective viral replication, an effective antiviral agent must prevent completion of the viral growth cycle in the infected cell without being toxic to the surrounding normal cells (Desselberger, 1995).

The proper choice of antiviral agent relies on the selectivity index (SI) that is calculated to be the ratio of cellular toxicity to antiviral potency *in vitro* (Snoeck *et al.*, 2002)

3. Definition and classification of antiviral agents

Antiviral drugs are a group of medication used for treatment of viral infections. It was formerly defined as substances other than a virus or virus containing vaccine or specific antibody which can produce either a protective or therapeutic effect to the clear detectable advantage of the virus infected host (Swallow, 1977).

Classification of antiviral agents is based on identification of a particular virus target for inhibition of a specific viral replication step.

3.1. Inhibitors of viral attachment/entry

Virus particles attach to the surface of host cells through an attachment site. Some viruses have specific attachment sites widely distributed all over the host cell membrane that recognize molecules on the surface of virus particle. This is followed by activation of an enzymatic activity that helps a change of the attachment site to allow entry of the virus into the cell. Different families of viruses have specific virus enzyme(s) whose action is to facilitate entry into the host cell. For example, the attachment site for myxoviruses is sialic acid and the virus enzyme is neuraminidase. Sometimes two different viruses share the same attachment/entry site e.g. Coxsackie and adenovirus receptor (CAR), but the way the individual virus utilize CAR differs.

Many viruses use heparan sulphate as an attachment site (Dunn and Spear, 1989). Other cell membrane surface proteins are used as receptors by different viruses: Cluster of differentiation molecules (e.g. CD4), members of immunoglobulin (Ig) superfamily, chemokine receptors (e.g. CXCR4), glycolipids, lipoproteins, transmembrane proteins (e.g. Claudins), scavenger proteins or tumor necrosis factor (TNF) superfamily proteins. Interactions between viral surface proteins and host cell plasma membrane molecules frequently result in conformational changes that increase the efficiency of virus endocytosis/ phagocytosis and virus-mediated pathogenicity.

Antiviral drugs may act by blocking the attachment process for specific viruses. Entry of HIV involves fusion between the viral lipid envelope and host plasma membrane. Fusion inhibitors can prevent HIV direct attachment and entry: Enfuvirtide (T-20) was the first approved viral entry inhibitor (Kilby and Eron, 2003). It inhibits fusion of HIV to cell by acting as a peptidomimetic that binds to the HIV gp41 envelope protein and thus preventing its attachment to CD4+ T cells. A circulating, highly specific natural HIV-1 inhibitor, designated virus-inhibitory peptide (VIRIP) was identified by Munch et al, (2007). VIRIP blocks HIV-1 entry by interacting with the gp41 fusion peptide and it was shown that a few amino acid changes increase its antiretroviral potency by two orders of magnitude. Maraviroc (UK-427,857) is a selective CCR5 cellular receptor antagonist with potent anti-HIV-1 activity (Dorr et al, 2005, Lieberman-Blum et al, 2008). It serves to intercept viral-host protein-protein interactions mediating entry (Friedrich et al, 2011).

St Vincent et al., (2010) showed that synthetic rigid amphipathic fusion inhibitors (RAFIs) inhibit the infectivity of several otherwise unrelated enveloped viruses, including hepatitis C virus (HCV) and HSV-1 and -2 with no cytotoxic or cytostatic effects (SI > 3,000) by inhibiting the increased negative curvature required for the initial stages of fusion. On the other hand, Wolf et al., (2010) reported LJ001 as a class of broad-spectrum antivirals effective against enveloped viruses that target the viral lipid membrane and compromises its ability to mediate virus-cell fusion. LJ001 specifically intercalated into viral membranes irreversibly, inactivated virions, while leaving functionally intact envelope proteins, and inhibited viral entry at a step after virus binding but before virus-cell fusion. Also, it was recently shown that the cellular Niemann-Pick C1-like 1 (NPC1L1) cholesterol uptake receptor is an HCV entry factor amendable to therapeutic intervention. Specifically, NPC1L1 expression is necessary for HCV infection, as silencing or antibody-mediated blocking of NPC1L1 impairs cell culture-derived HCV (HCVcc) infection initiation (Sainz et al., 2012)

The second step in viral replication cycle is penetration. Enveloped viruses penetrate by fusion of the viral membrane with the cell membrane (fusion from without); however, naked viruses penetrate the cell by phagocytosis of the virion from the extracellular fluid (fusion from within). Among antiviral agents that inhibit fusion are pooled immunoglobulin, hyperimmune serum & Enfuvirtide (T-20).

3.2. Inhibitors of virus uncoating and virus genome release

In the cytoplasm cellular and virus proteases become activated by the acidic pH created inside the phagosome /endocytosome sac.Proteolytic digestion of virus capsid (naked viruses) or virus envelope (enveloped viruses) ends by complete release of virus genetic nucleoproteins.

The viral genome is released and activated by several mechanisms specific to virus families. The details are much but the end result is the start of virus replication.

Rimantadine and Amantadine specifically prevent uncoating of Influenza A (not B) virus. This is achieved by binding to virus protein M2 and blocking its action as a proton ion channel that allows acidification of the virus core needed for activation of viral RNA transcriptase. In some strains, it may inhibit virus assembly.

Amantadine is the 1-amino derivative of adamantine a complex 10- carbon compound with a cage-like structure and rimantadine is a nearly identical methyl derivative of amantadine (Hirsch et al, 1996).

Characterization of the three-dimensional structure of picornaviruses in the 1980s allowed the development of compounds targeted at the virus itself (Florea et al, 2003). Pleconaril is known to be a broad spectrum anti-picornaviral agent that binds to a hydrophobic pocket in the viral capsid inducing conformational changes, which lead to altered receptor binding and viral uncoating (Romero, 2001). Pleconaril was designed to bind the highly conserved hydrophobic binding site on VP1 protein of Picorna viruses (Hussain Basha and Prasad, 2012). Clinical studies have reported a reduction in the duration and intensity of symptoms in children and adults with enteroviral meningitis and in adults with rhinoviral respiratory tract infections treated with pleconaril. Also, pleconaril has demonstrated efficacy in the treatment of severe life-threatening enteroviral infections of the newborn and in immunosuppressed individuals. (Romero, 2001).

3.3. Inhibitors of virus replication

"All RNA viruses replicate in the cytoplasm except paramyxo viruses and retroviruses and all DNA viruses replicate in the nucleus solely except pox viruses."

RNA viruses with + ve RNA single strand genome that can act directly as virus mRNA e.g. polioviruses and hepatitis C virus use common " cellular" machines for synthesis of virus protein termed internal ribosome entry site (IRES) – mediated translation. This system of translation initiation involves entry of 40 S ribosome internally to the 5′ untranslated region (UTR) of viral RNA by a cap- independent translation using specific virus initiation factors and IRES elements required for IRES mediated translation. Because there is no RNA polymerase proofing system, several mutations occur during new viral RNA genome formation leading to quasispecies of viral RNA genome.

DNA viruses produce viral mRNA transcripts soon after the infection of a cell through host –cell enzyme, DNA dependent RNA polymerase II. DNA virus replication is semi conservative and is very accurate since DNA polymerase checks the copied sequences (proofreading) and removes any mismatch.

3.3.1. Polymerase inhibitors

Acyclovir and other antiherpes nucleoside and nucleotide analog drugs; (Identified by the suffix –cyclovir/ -ciclovir"); Valacyclovir, Famciclovir, Penciclovir, Ganciclovir, Cidofovir (cytosine analogue). These agents interfere with virus replication and spread to new neighbouring cells by selective inhibition of an enzyme, thymidine kinase (TK) that the virus has but human cells do not, and thus interrupting the virus capability to synthesize its own DNA (table 2).CMV and EBV encode their own TK. HSV, VZV and EBV encoded TKs catalyze the phosphorylation of acyclovir to acyclovir monophosphate (ACVMP), as well as of thymidine and some other nucleoside analogue to their respective monophosphate. The markedly selective action of Acyclovir against HSV-1, HSV-2 and VZV is a consequence of several enzymatic reactions, each of which is unique for virus replication; 1) Specific activation by a virus induced TK into ACVMP, which is converted by cellular kinases to acyclovir di- and triphosphate (ACVTP), the metabolically active form of acyclovir. 2) Selective inhibition of the viral DNA polymerase by ACVTP acting as a competitor with dGTP 3) termination of viral DNA chain elongation by incorporation of ACVMP (Hirsch et al, 1996)and 4) inactivation of the viral DNA polymerase following ACVMP incorporation in the presence of dNTPs (Reardon& Spector, 1992). Also, 2-chloro-3-pyridin-3-yl-5, 6, 7, 8-tetrahydroindolizine-1-carboxamide (CMV423), showed very potent *in vitro* activity against human cytomegalovirus (HCMV). It acts on a step of the viral replicative cycle that precedes the DNA polymerase step and, most likely, coincides with the immediate early (IE) antigen synthesis (Snoeck et al, 2002).It also acts against human herpes viruses (HHV) HHV-6, and HHV-7 at low concentrations, but shows only modest activity against herpes simplex virus (HSV) HSV-1 and -2 and none against varicella-zoster virus (VZV) (Snoeck *et al.*, 2002; De Bolle, 2004).

Telbivudine (LdT) is a synthetic thymidine nucleoside analogue. It is used to treat hepatitis B viral infection. It acts by blocking Viral DNA polymerase activity. Clinical trials demonstrated that telbivudine is safe and potent antiviral agent for treatment of chronic hepatitis B .It has superior efficacy compared to lamivudine(3TC) and adefovir (Lui and Chan,2008) Systematic review and meta-analysis of clinical trials showed that LdT is superior in inhibiting HBV replication and preventing drug resistance as compared to 3TC for CHB patients (Zhao et al, 2010). Adefovir(ADV) (Leung, 2005), Tenofovir and Entecavir are also nucleoside analogues with anti-HBV activity. They competitively inhibit HBV DNA polymerase ending in viral DNA chain termination after replacing viral nucleosides.

3.3.2. Nucleoside reverse transcriptase inhibitors (NRTIs)

This group includes antiviral agents that are mainly recognized for the treatment of HIV, usually in combination with other retroviral drugs (Table 3). NRTIs are the first agents that were entered into clinical trials and received approval for treatment of HIV infection (Patick & Potts, 1998).

Drug	Chemical structure	Viruses	Target
Acyclovir	Synthetic acyclic guanosine analogue [9(2hydroxyethoxymethyl)guanine] TK activated	herpes simplex virus types 1 and 2, varicella zoster virus (VZV)	viral DNA polymerase
Ganciclovir	Nucleoside analogue (acyclic analogue of guanosine) that have an extra hydroxyl methyl group on the acyclic side chain. 9-(1,3-dihydroxy- 2-propoxymethyl)guanine) virus UL97 gene-specified kinase activated (Mims et al, 2006)	Herpes viruses especially CMV	viral DNA polymerase
Cidofovir	Nucleotide analogue (S)-1-(3-hydroxy2phosphonylmethoxypropyl)cytosine) Not TK activated	CMV, HSV, Adenovirus Papillomavirus	viral DNA polymerase
Vidarbine	Nucleoside analogue (adenine) (9-β-D-ribofuranosyladenine) Not TK activated	HSV,VZV, (less effective against CMV & EBV), poxviruses, rhabdoviruses, hepadnaviruses	viral DNA polymerase
Idoxuridine	Nucleoside analogue- iodinated thymidine. Replaces thymidine in the DNA -- blocks further elongation. Virus K activated	Herpes viruses & other DNA viruses	viral DNA polymerase
Foscarnet	Non nucleoside analogue (pyrophosphate analogue); phosphonoformic acid, trisodium salt. Not TK activated	cytomegalovirus (CMV) and herpes simplex viruses types 1 and 2 (HSV-1 and HSV-2	viral DNA polymerase and HIV reverse transcriptase

Table 2. Common viral DNA polymerase inhibitors

Zidovudine

Zidovudine (azidothymidine) is a synthetic pyrimidine analogue. It is an analogue of the nucleoside thymidine in which the hydroxyl group on the ribose is replaced by an azido group (Hirsch et al, 1996). After conversion to the triphosphate by cellular enzymes, it acts as a competitive inhibitor of, and substrate for the viral reverse transcriptase. The azido group prevents the formation of phosphodiester linkages. Proviral DNA formation is blocked because AZT triphosphate is incorporated into the DNA with resulting chain termination (Mims et al, 2006, Chapter 33).

Drug	Chemical Name	Target Viruses
Zidovudine*(AZT; ZDV)	Azidothymidine	HIV
Stavudine*(d4T)	2′,3′didehydro-3′-deoxythymidine	HIV
Zalcitabine*(ddC)	2′,3′- dideoxycytidine	HIV
Lamivudine*(3TC)	dideoxy-thiacytidine analogue	HIV Hepatitis B
emtricitabine(Emtriva)*	Deoxycytidine nucleoside analogue	HIV
Didanosine*(ddI)	2′,3′- dideoxyinosine	HIV
Abacavir (ABC)	nucleoside analog reverse transcriptase inhibitor	HIV
Tenofovir**(Tenofovir DF)	an acyclic nucleoside phosphonate (nucleotide) analog of adenosine 5'-monophosphate	HIV

* All are recognized by the "INE" suffix

** Tenofovir is a nucleoTide reverse transcriptase inhibitor

Table 3. Common Nucleoside Reverse Transcriptase Inhibitors

Lamivudine (3TC)

Lamivudine is a dideoxy-thiacytidine analogue with potent antiviral property against hepatitis B virus (Leung, 2005).Lamivudine acts as a nucleoside inhibitor of reverse transcriptase.It inhibits HBV reverse transcriptase, blocks the completion of the double stranded circular DNA before migration to the cell nucleus and prevents the infection of new hepatocytes. However, Lamivudine resistance developed after five years of monotherapy.

Tenofovir (TDF)

Tenofovir is a new nucleoside analogue with selective activity against hepatitis B virus. It was licensed in 2008 for the treatment of HBV infections in Europe and the United States (Schooley et al, 2002, Zhao et al, 2011). It is active against wild type and Lamivudine resistant HBV, both *in vitro* (Lada et al, 2004) and *in vivo* (Lacombe et al, 2005).

Systematic review and meta-analysis of clinical trials was conducted by Zhao et al (2011) to compare the efficacy of tenofovir and adefovir in the treatment of chronic hepatitis B. Meta-analysis indicated that a twelve-month TDF treatment was superior to ADV in inhibiting HBV replication in CHB patients. But there was no significant difference in the ALT normalization, HBeAg seroconversion and HBsAg loss rate.

3.3.3. Non nucleosides reverse transcriptase inhibitors (NNRTI)

Travertine, Delavirdine, Efavirenz, Nevirapine.

These drugs directly bind to different sites in the reverse transcriptase (RT) enzyme and prevent its action. They do not require phosphorylation for activation and do not compete with nucleoside triphosphates.

3.3.4. Inhibitors of RNA synthesis (RNA polymerase inhibitors)

Ribavirin: It is a synthetic purine nucleoside derivative- that resembles guanosine. Ribavirin inhibits guanosine triphosphate formation, prevents capping of viral mRNA, and blocks viral RNA-dependent RNA polymerase activity (Hirsch et al, 1996). It has got a broad spectrum antiviral activity as it inhibits replication of many DNA and RNA viruses such as HCV, Influenza A and B, parainfluenza, respiratory syncytial virus (RSV), paramyxovirus and HIV.

The combination of Interferon alpha/Ribavirin therapy was approved by the United States regulatory authorities in 1998. The clinical efficacy of this combination exceeds that of the summation of individual monotherapies (Lau et al, 2002).Four mechanisms of action of ribavirin in HCV therapy were proposed. The first line of action consists of 2 possible indirect mechanisms: (1) enhancement of host T-cell–mediated immunity against viral infection through switching the T-cell phenotype from type 2 to type 1 and (2) inhibition of the host enzyme inosine monophosphate dehydrogenase (IMPDH). The second line of action consists of 2 other hypotheses: (1) direct inhibition of HCV RNA, including NS5B-encoded RNA dependent RNA polymerase (RdRp) and (2) as an RNA mutagen that drives a rapidly mutating RNA virus over the threshold to "error catastrophe." (Lau et al, 2002).

On the other hand, specifically targeted antiviral therapy for hepatitis C (STAT-C) will probably supplement or replace present therapies. Leading compounds for STAT-C target the HCV nonstructural (NS) 5B polymerase and NS3 protease and helicase domain of the HCV NS3 protein (Belon and Frick, 2009).

3.4. Inhibitors of viral protein synthesis

All viruses use the cellular ribosomes to translate their viral mRNA. The later is translated into the structural proteins that will constitute core, envelope proteins and viral enzymes. As an example, the Enteroviruses (EV) RNA genome directs the synthesis of a single polyprotein that is autocatalytically processed into mature proteins at Gln ↓Gly cleavage sites by the 3C protease (3Cpro), which has narrow, conserved substrate specificity. These cleavages are essential for virus replication, making 3Cpro an excellent target for antivirus drug development (Costenaro et al, 2011). The crystal structure of 3Cpro from an enterovirus B, EV-93, a recently identified pathogen, alone and in complex with the anti-HRV molecules compound 1 (AG7404) and rupintrivir (AG7088) was determined by Costenaro et al (2011). They found that the EV-93 3Cpro adopts a chymotrypsin-like fold with a canonically configured oxyanion hole and a substrate binding pocket similar to that of rhino-, coxsackie- and poliovirus 3C proteases (Costenaro et al, 2011). Collectively, neuraminidase enzyme regulates the synthesis of viral and cell membrane glycoprotein during Influenza virus A and B replication, which characterizes the enzyme as a target of viral protein modification inhibitors (neuraminidase inhibitors).

Other examples of viral proteins synthesis inhibitors are Fomivirsen and Interferon. Fomivirsen is an oligonucleotide that binds to CMV mRNA and blocks its replication and thus inhibits the synthesis of proteins that are essential for production of infectious CMV. It is a potent and selective antiviral agent for cytomegalovirus retinitis (Geary et al, 2002). Interferons are a group of virus induced proteins that interrupts new viral protein formation by several mechanisms .They possess direct complex intracellular antiviral, antiproliferative, and immunomodulating activities (Lau et al, 2002). IFN-α and -β have got antiviral activity whereas IFN-γ is predominantly immunomodulatory. rIFN-α and rIFN-β are approved for treatment of HCV, HBV, HPV and HHV-8 (Kaposi sarcoma) infections.

Gene targeting studies have distinguished four main effector pathways of the IFN-mediated antiviral response: the Mx GTPase pathway, the 2', 5'-oligoadenylate-synthetase-directed ribonuclease L pathway, the protein kinase R pathway and the ISG15 ubiquitin-like pathway. These effectors pathways individually block viral transcription, degrade viral RNA, inhibit translation and modify protein function to control all steps of viral replication (Sadler &Williams, 2008).

The aim of HCV/ HBV treatment is to develop a sustained decline of viral load by inhibition of viral replication, allowing CTL-derived cytokines to reduce the number of hepatocytes supporting viral replication by direct killing and also improvement of liver histopathology by the decline of HBV/HCV infected hepatocytes This will decrease fibrosis and hepatocytes regeneration with subsequent reduction of liver cirrhosis and thus prevention of progression to hepatocellular carcinoma.

As suggested by Sainz et al, (2012), optimal HCV therapy will probably require a combination of antiviral targeting multiple aspects of the viral lifecycle. Recently, high rate of sustained virologic response was achieved when two direct-acting antiviral agents (NS5A replication complex inhibitor daclatasvir and the NS3 protease inhibitor asunaprevir) were combined with peginterferon alfa-2a and ribavirin for treatment of HCV chronic hepatitis patients (Lok et al, 2012).

Several drugs are recommended for treatment of patients with chronic hepatitis B (CHB).These anti HBV drugs are used to compose combinational therapy with the addition of interferon sometimes to delay drug resistance. These drugs can be divided into two main groups based on their mechanism of action, namely immunomodulatory drugs like alpha interferons and antiviral drugs including lamivudine(LAM), telbivudine(LdT), entecavir(ETV), adefovir(ADV), and tenofovir(TDF) (Zhao et al, 2011).Interferon and Lamivudine have been the only approved agents for a while. The approval of Adefovir in 2002, Pegylated Interferons and Entecavir in 2005 opens up more choices and chances (Leung, 2005).

3.4.1. Protease inhibitors (PIs): (inhibit the post-translational events)

Various drugs recognized by "NAVIR" suffix are known to have the same mode of action; *Amprenavir, Saquinavir, Darunavir, Atazanavir, Ritonavir, Tipranavir Indinavir, Nelfinavir.*

This group of drugs acts by preventing the activity of cellular/viral proteases enzymes. Proteases are valid targets for antiviral agents as they are essential for the production of mature infectious virus particles. Molecular studies have indicated that viral proteases play a critical role in the life cycle of many viruses by affecting the cleavage of high-molecular-weight viral polyprotein precursors to yield functional products or by catalyzing the processing of the structural proteins necessary for assembly and morphogenesis of virus particles (Patick & Potts, 1998).

Several studies elaborated the value of protease inhibitors for the treatment of a lot of RNA and DNA viruses; HIV, HCV, Picorna viruses, RSV, Herpes viruses, Rota virus & severe acute respiratory syndrome virus (SARS). HIV protease inhibitors have emerged as potent antiretroviral chemotherapeutic agents that, in combination with RTIs, have resulted in prolonged suppression of viral replication (Patick & Potts, 1998). Also, in HCV treatment, direct acting antivirals (DAA), in clinical development include NS3-4A protease inhibitors (two of which, telaprevir and boceprevir, have recently been approved for treatment of HCV genotype 1 infection in combination with pegylated interferon-α and ribavirin (Pawlotsky, 2012). Replication of picornaviruses and coronaviruses requires 3Cpro (3C protease) and 3CLpro (3C-like protease) respectively, which are structurally analogous (Ramajayam et al, 2011). A group of common inhibitors against 3C (pro) and 3CL (pro) were found recently (Wang and Liang, 2010).

3.4.2. Integrase inhibitor: Raltegravir

Integrase is an essential HIV-1-specific enzyme that is an active target for antiretroviral drug development. The drug specifically inhibits strand transfer, one of the three steps of HIV integration into the host DNA (Katlama and Murphy, 2009) and thus prevents human immunodeficiency virus from multiplying in the host.

Inhibition of HIV replication initially targeted viral enzymes, which are exclusively expressed by the virus and not present in the human cell (Sierra-Aragón and Walter, 2012).

Table 4 illustrates Common FDA approved antiviral agents for the treatment of HIV infection (www.fda.gov/.../hivandaidsactivities/ucm118915.ht.)

Analogue to HCV therapy, combination therapy for treatment of HIV reduces HIV replication with subsequent drop in viral load. Two NRTIs in combination with the NNRTI or PI drugs have had a dramatic effect on progression to AIDS and led to the term Highly Active Anti-Retroviral Therapy (HAART) (Mims et al, 2006- chapter 21). The combination includes:

Nucleoside/ Nucleotides Reverse Transcriptase Inhibitors (NRTIs) such as Tenofovir and Abacavir

Non-Nucleoside/ Nucleotides Reverse Transcriptase Inhibitors (NNRTIs) such as Efavirenz and Nevirapine

Integrase Inhibitors such as Raltegravir

Protease Inhibitors (PIs) such as Darunavir and Atazanavir

Fusion and Entry Inhibitors such as Enfuvirtide and Maraviroc.

Name	Mechanism of action
Lamivudine,zidovudine,emtricitabine, abacavir, stavudine,didanosine, zalcitabine	Nucleoside Reverse Transcriptase Inhibitors (NRTIs)
tenofovir disoproxil fumarate	Nucleotide reverse transcriptase inhibitor (NtRTI)
Rilpivirine,delavirdine,etravirine,efavirenz, nevirapine,nevirapine	Nonnucleoside Reverse Transcriptase Inhibitors (NNRTIs)
Amprenavir, tipranavir, lopinavir (combined with ritonavir at a 4/1 ratio),indinavir,ritonavir,darunavir, nelfinavir, atazanavir	Protease Inhibitors (PIs)
enfuvirtide, T-20	Fusion Inhibitors
maraviroc	Entry Inhibitors - CCR5 co-receptor antagonist
raltegravir	integrase inhibitors

(www.fda.gov/.../hivandaidsactivities/ucm118915.ht.)

Table 4. Common FDA approved antiviral agents for the treatment of HIV infection

3.5. Inhibitors of viral exit (release)

Viral release is done by single burst releasing millions of new viral particles from infected cells or by slow process of budding through the plasma membrane allowing the infected cell to survive for several days while supporting viral replication and release. In general, lytic viruses (e.g: polio) are released by lysis and death of the cell. Others (e.g. influenza, HIV, and measles) escape by budding from the cell surface.

3.5.1. Neuraminidase inhibitors

Oseltamivir and Zanamivir are antivirals used to treat and prevent influenza (Jefferson et al, 2012). They Inhibit neuraminidases produced by influenza A and B (enzyme which cleaves the interaction between sialic acid cell surface receptors and viral proteins and surface proteins of infected cells and thus allow for release of virions) Therefore, these drugs interfere with the release of influenza virus from infected host cells.

Table 5 sums up antivirals that are available commercially, used by physicians and approved by international and national regulatory authorities.

Virus	Anti-Viral Drugs
Human immunodeficiency virus	22 approved agents
Hepatitis C virus	pegIFN, Ribavirin
Hepatitis B virus	Interferon-alpha (pegylated), Lamivudine, adefovir
Herpesviruses	Acyclovir,famciclovir,valacyclovir,ganciclovir, cidofovir, formivirsen,valganciclovir
Influenza	Amantadine, rimantadine,zanamivir, oseltamivir
Respiratory syncytial virus	Ribavirin, Palivizumab
Picornaviruses	pleconaril
Papillomaviruses	IFN(intra-lesional), ?cidofovir, Fluorouracil
Rhinoviruses	Tremacamra (rsICAM-1)

Table 5. Master Anti-Viral Drugs

4. Antiviral from plants

Plants and plants extracts have been used chiefly as traditional medicine for centuries even before the active principles in the plant products could be elucidated through the improvements in science and technology. The World Health Organisation (WHO) has estimated that perhaps 80% of the world's population rely on traditional medicine for the treatment of infectious diseases (Abonyi et al, 2009).

Several naturally occurring dietary flavonoids including quercetin, hesperetin, and catechin were previously studied *in vitro* in cell culture monolayers using viral plaque reduction technique and proved to be effective on the infectivity and replication of HSV-1, poliovirus type 1, parainfluenza virus type 3 (Pf-3), and respiratory syncytial virus (RSV). Quercetin caused a concentration-dependent reduction in the infectivity of each virus. Hesperetin had no effect on infectivity but it reduced intracellular replication of each of the viruses. Catechin inhibited the infectivity but not the replication of RSV and HSV-1 and had negligible effects on the other viruses (Kaul et al, 1985).

We previously had the opportunity to evaluate extracts of five different herbal plants for hepatitis A (HAV) antiviral activities by plaque reduction assay. These plants were anise, chamomile, liquorice, nigella and thyme. A fast growing HAV-10 reported to be cytopathic for *Vero* cell culture was used where the plant extracts were screened for anti-infective, protection and antireplicative activities. The rates of the anti-infection studies were arranged in a decreasing order as follows: anise> liquorice > chamomile > thyme>. The rates of the protective antiviral activities were found to be as follows: chamomile >liquorice> thyme > anise. The rate of the anti-replication effect was ordered in the following decreasing order: thyme > liquorice > chamomile > nigella. Thus anise extract was devoid of any anti-replication activity, whereas nigella extract was devoid of any protective activity against HAV infection i*n vitro* (Omran et al, 2001)

Also, another Egyptian study evaluated the antiviral activities of the essential oils of the fresh leaves of 3 *Melaleuca* species; *M. ericifolia, M. leucadendron,* and *M. armillaris* against *Herpes simplex virus* type 1 (HSV-1) in African green monkey kidney cells (Vero) by a plaque reduction assay. It was found that the volatile oil of *M. armillaris* was more effective as a virucidal (up to 99%) than that of *M. leucadendron* (92%) and *M. ericifolia* (91.5%) (Farag et al, 2004).

Amylose extracted from Grateloupia filicina have antivirus activity in the stage of HSV-2 binding, adsorption and ingression with Vero cell (Zhu et al, 2006).

Also, it was shown by Verma et al, (2009) that Picroliv or Kutkin of Picrorhiza kurroa which constitute an important component of many Indian herbal preparations has anti-viral and immune-stimulant activities.

Screening of the antiviral activity of oil extract of Balanites aegyptiaca (Balantiaceae) fruits against Herpes simplex virus type -1 in African green monkey kidney cells (Vero) by a plaque reduction assay, illustrated that the oil had virucidal activity (58.3%) against Herpes simplex virus type 1 at concentration 50μg/ml compared with acyclovir (60%) at the same concentration (Al Ashaal et al, 2010).

The antiviral activity of Balanites aegyptiaca herb was also reported against HIV/AIDS (Chaudhry and Khoo, 2004).

We also have the experience of testing extracts from Egyptian medical plants for their potential antiviral activity at different stages of viral replication. The anti-influenza activity of hydro-alcoholic extracts from; Cleome droserifolia, Justicia ghiesbreghtiana, and Thunbergia grandiflora against a fast growing Influenza "A" reference strain (H3N2) in replicating Madin–Darby Canine kidney (MDCK) was performed. Amantadine was used as reference anti-influenza virus drug. Three antiviral assays were used; Anti-infectivity, protective and anti-replication mechanisms, reduction in the number of plaques formed by the virus in MDCK cells treated with maximum non toxic dose (MNTD) of each plant extract was analyzed. Justicia extract showed the highest significant inhibition of influenza virus infectivity .On the other hand, when MDCK cells were pretreated with cleome extract for 48 hours before infection with influenza virus, it showed the highest significant anti-influenza virus activity. Whereas, when cleome extract was added to MDCK infected with influenza virus after 60 min of infection, it induced significant inhibition in influenza virus type A replication in a dose dependent relation. Thunbergia extract had the least antiviral activity. Phytochemical screening tests showed that all of the studied extracts contain tannins but flavonoids are present in the Cleome and Justicia extracts only. Two major compounds of cleome extract; Isorhamnetin-3-0-B glucopyranosyl-7-0 -L-rhamnopyranoside and quercetin -3-0-B – glucopyranosly-7-0-L rhamnopyranoside were studied for their antiviral activity by the three different assays. The results proved that isorhamnetin produced inhibition of influenza virus infectivity stronger than that produced by the total cleome extract (Elkosy et al, 2005).

Antiviral activity of dandelion extracts against influenza viruses was reported by Wen et al, (2011). Mechanisms of reduction of viral growth in MDCK or A549 cells by dandelion involve inhibition of virus replication. Dandelion extracts inhibited infections in Madin-Darby canine kidney (MDCK) cells or Human lung adenocarcinoma cell line (A549) of PR8 or WSN viruses, as well as inhibited polymerase activity and reduced virus nucleoprotein (NP) RNA level. The plant extract did not exhibit any apparent negative effects on cell viability, metabolism or proliferation at the effective dose (Wen et al, 2011).

In general, the medicinal plants are potential antiviral agents that are locally available, relatively cheap, can be tested for safety and non toxicity and culturally acceptable to the community.

5. Conclusions

Potent antiviral agents are on the increase leading to improved patient management. Viruses replicate inside live nucleated cells in different steps using cellular machinery, but sometimes virus specific enzymes are used. This allows for the selection of virus specific molecules as targets of antivirals. An effective antiviral therapy depends greatly on its ability to block viral entry or viral exit from infected cell or inhibiting active viral replication steps. Proper understanding of these steps at molecular level and the use of advanced *in silico* design for development of antivirals that specifically react with viral target molecule may provide new insight for their potential activity and prophylaxis against viral infections.

Author details

Zeinab N. Said and Kouka S. Abdelwahab
Faculty of Medicine (for Girls)-Al-Azhar University, Cairo, Egypt

6. References

Abonyi, D. O., Adikwu, M. U., Esimone, C. O. and Ibezim, E. C. (2009) Plants as sources of antiviral agents. *African Journal of Biotechnology;* 8 (17): 3989-3994 ISSN: 1684-5315

Al Ashaal H A, Farghaly A A, Abd El Aziz M.M, Ali M.A. (2010) Phytochemical investigation and medicinal evaluation of fixed oil of Balanites aegyptiaca fruits (Balantiaceae). *Journal of Ethnopharmacology;* 127(2), Feb.: 495–501

Belon CA, Frick DN. (2009) Helicase inhibitors as specifically targeted antiviral therapy for hepatitis C. Future Virol. 1; 4(3) May: 277-293. PMID: 20161209

Chaudhry T.M, Khoo C.S. (2004) Balanites Herbs Potential Remedy for HIV/AIDS and Other Ailments, vol. 47. Hamdard Medicus, Bait al-Hikmah, Karachi, Pakistan, pp. 42–44.

Costenaro L, Kaczmarska Z, Arnan C, Janowski R, Coutard B, Solà M, Gorbalenya A, Norder H, Canard B, and Coll M (2011) Structural Basis for Antiviral Inhibition of the Main Protease, 3C, from Human Enterovirus 93. *J Virol.*; 85: 10764–10773.

DeBolle, Andrei G., Snoeck R., Zhang Y, Van Lommel A, Otto M, Bousseau A, Roy C, De Clercq E, Naesens L. (2004) Potent, selective and cell-mediated inhibition of human herpesvirus 6 at an early stage of viral replication by the non-nucleoside compound CMV423. *Biochem. Pharmacol.*; 67 (2), Jan.:325–336. PMID: 14698045

De Clercq E. (2001). Molecular targets for antiviral agents. *J Pharmacol Exp Ther.*; 297(1), Apr: 1-10.

Desselberger U (1995) Molecular Epidermiology, In: *Medical Virology*: A Practical Approach. Desselberger U (ed) Oxford University Press, New York, pp. 173-190.

Dorr P, Westby M, Dobbs S, Griffin P, Irvine B, Macartney M, Mori J, Rickett G, Smith-Burchnell C, Napier C, Webster R, Armour D, Price D, Stammen B, Wood A, Perros M.(2005)Maraviroc (UK-427,857), a potent, orally bioavailable, and selective small-molecule inhibitor of chemokine receptor CCR5 with broad-spectrum anti-human immunodeficiency virus type 1 activity. *Antimicrob Agents Chemother.*;49(11):4721-32.

Dunn Wu and Spear P G. (1989).Initial interaction of herpes simplex virus with cells is binding to heparan sulfate. *Journal of Virology*: 63 (1): 52-58

El-kosy RH, Ismail LD, El-Gendy OD, Said ZN & Abdel-Wahab KS. (2005) Phytomedicine: Anti Influenza A virus activity of three herbal extracts. *Egyptian Journal of Virology* 2(1):21-39

Farag R. S., Shalaby A. S., El-Baroty G. A., Ibrahim N. A., Ali M. A. And Hassan E. M. (2004) Chemical and biological evaluation of the essential oils of different Melaleuca species. *Phytother. Res.* 18(1), Jan.: 30–35 DOI: 10.1002/ptr.1348.

Florea NR, Maglio D, Nicolau DP.(2003) Pleconaril, a novel antipicornaviral agent. *Pharmacotherapy.* 2003 Mar;23(3):339-48.

Friedrich BM, Dziuba N, Li G, Endsley MA, Murray JL, Ferguson MR (2011). Host factors mediating HIV-1 replication. *Virus Res.* Nov;161(2):101-14.Geary RS, Henry SP, Grillone LR. (2002) Fomivirsen: clinical pharmacology and potential drug interactions. *Clin Pharmacokinet.*; 41(4):255-60.

Hirsch MS, Kaplan JC and D' Aquila RT (1996) Antiviral agents In: *Fields Virology (volume 1) - third edition,* Fields BR, Knipe DM, Howley PM, pp: 431-466, Lippincott – Raven, ISBN 0-7817-0253-4, Philadelphia-New York

Hussain Basha S, Prasad RN.(2012) In-Silico screening of Pleconaril and its novel substituted derivatives with Neuraminidase of H1N1 Influenza strain. *BMC Res Notes.* Feb 17;5:105.

Jefferson T, Jones MA, Doshi P, Del Mar CB, Heneghan CJ, Hama R, Thompson MJ. (2012)Neuraminidase inhibitors for preventing and treating influenza in healthy adults and children. *Cochrane Database of Systematic Reviews*; Jan 18; 1: CD008965.PMID:22258996 [PubMed - in process]

Katlama C, Murphy R. (2009)Emerging role of integrase inhibitors in the management of treatment-experienced patients with HIV infection. *Ther Clin Risk Manag.*; 5(2) Apr: 331-40. PMID: 19536321

Kaul TN, Middleton E Jr, Ogra PL. (1985)Antiviral effect of flavonoids on human viruses. *J Med Virol.*; 15(1) Jan.:71-9. PMID: 2981979

Kilby JM, Eron JJ. (2003) Novel therapies based on mechanisms of HIV-1 cell entry. *N Engl J Med*. May 348(22):2228-38 Review.PMID:12773651

Lada O, Benhamou Y, Cahour A, Katlama C, Poynard T, Thibault V (2004) In vitro susceptibility of lamivudine-resistant hepatitis B virus to adefovir and tenofovir. *Antivir Ther*, 9:353-363.

Lacombe K, Gozlan J, Boelle PY, Serfaty L, Zoulim F, Valleron AJ, Girard PM (2005)Long-term hepatitis B virus dynamics in HIV-hepatitis B virus-co-infected patients treated with tenofovir disoproxil fumarate. *AIDS*, 19:907-915.

Lau JY, Tam RC, Liang TJ, Hong Z. (2002)Mechanism of action of ribavirin in the combination treatment of chronic HCV infection. *Hepatology.*; 35(5): May: 1002-9.

Leung N. (2005) Comparison of lamividine and adefovir dipivoxil in the treatment of chronic hepatitis B. *Hep B Annual*; 2(1):93-126

Lieberman-Blum SS, Fung HB, Bandres JC. (2008) Maraviroc: a CCR5-receptor antagonist for the treatment of HIV-1 *infection Clin Ther.*; 30(7):1228-50.

Lok AS, Gardiner DF, Lawitz E, Martorell C, Everson GT, Ghalib R, Reindollar R, Rustgi V, McPhee F, Wind-Rotolo M, Persson A, Zhu K, Dimitrova DI, Eley T, Guo T, Grasela DM, Pasquinelli C. (2012)Preliminary study of two antiviral agents for hepatitis C genotype 1. *N Engl J Med.* 19; 366(3) Jan.:216-24. PMID: 22256805

Lorizate M, Kräusslich HG. (2011)Role of lipids in virus replication. *Cold Spring Harb Perspect Biol.* 1; 3(10) Oct.:a004820. PMID: 21628428

Lui YY, Chan HL. (2008) A review of telbivudine for the management of chronic hepatitis B virus infection. *Expert Opin Drug Metab Toxicol.*; 4(10) Oct: 1351-61. PMID: 18798704

Mims C, Dockrell HM, G RV, Roitt I, Wakelin D & Zuckerman M.2006. Chapter 21; Sexually transmitted diseases; page 270-272 In *Medical Microbiology* (Updated Third Edition).Elsevier ISBN: 0 7234 3403 4, Spain

Mims C, Dockrell HM, G RV, Roitt I, Wakelin D & Zuckerman M.2006 Chapter 33; Attacking the enemy: antimicrobial agents and chemotherapy; page 473-51 In *Medical Microbiology*(UpdatedThird Edition).Elsevier ISBN:0 7234 3403 4, Spain

Münch J, Ständker L, Adermann K, Schulz A, Schindler M, Chinnadurai R, Pöhlmann S, Chaipan C, Biet T, Peters T, Meyer B, Wilhelm D, Lu H, Jing W, Jiang S, Forssmann WG, Kirchhoff F. (2007) Discovery and optimization of a natural HIV-1 entry inhibitor targeting the gp41 fusion peptide. *Cell.* 20; 129(2) April: 263-75. PMID: 17448989

Omran ME, Mohamed TR, ZN. Said, Abdel-Wahab KS. Ashour MS. (2001) Investigation of anti hepatitis A activities of five medical plants used in folk medicine.AZ. *J. Microbiol*; 51 Jan.: 54-71

Patick A. K. and Potts K. E. (1998) Protease Inhibitors as Antiviral Agents. *Clin Microbiol Rev.*; 11(4) Oct: 614-627 PMID: 9767059

Pawlotsky JM. (2012) New antiviral agents for hepatitis C. F1000 *Biol Rep.*;4:5. Epub Mar 1PMID:22403588

Ramajayam R, Tan KP, Liang PH. (2011) Recent development of 3C and 3CL protease inhibitors for anti-coronavirus and anti-picornavirus drug discovery. *Biochem Soc Trans.*; 39(5) Oct: 1371-5. PMID: 21936817

Reardon JE& Spector T. (1992) Acyclovir: mechanism of antiviral action and potentiatiion by ribonucleotide reductase inhibitors. *ADVPharacol*; 22: 1-27

Romero JR.(2001) Pleconaril: a novel antipicornaviral drug. *Expert Opin Investig Drugs.* Feb;10(2):369-79.

Sadler, A.J. &Williams, B.R.G. (2008) interferon-inducible antiviral effectors. *Nature Reviews Immunology* 8: July: 559-568 doi: 10.1038/nri2314.

Sainz B Jr, Barretto N, Martin DN, Hiraga N, Imamura M, Hussain S, Marsh KA, Yu X, Chayama K, Alrefai WA, Uprichard SL. (2012) Identification of the Niemann-Pick C1-like 1 cholesterol absorption receptor as a new hepatitis C virus entry factor. *Nat Med.* 8; 18(2) Jan.:281-5. PMID: 22231557

Schooley RT, Ruane P, Myers RA, Beall G, Lampiris H, Berger D, Chen SS, Miller MD, Isaacson E, Cheng AK.(2002)Tenofovir DF in antiretroviral-experienced patients: results from a 48-week, randomized, double-blind study. *AIDS*, 16:1257-1263.

Sierra-Aragón S, Walter H (2012). Targets for inhibition of HIV replication: entry, enzyme action, release and maturation. *Intervirology.*;55(2):84-97.

Snoeck R, Andrei G, Bodaghi B, Lagneaux L, Daelemans D, de Clercq E, Neyts J, Schols D, Naesens L, Michelson S, Bron D, Otto MJ, Bousseau A, Nemecek C, RoyC. (2002).2-Chloro-3-pyridin-3-yl-5, 6, 7, 8-tetrahydroindolizine-1-carboxamide (CMV423), a new lead compound for the treatment of human cytomegalovirus infections. *Antiviral Res.*; 55(3) Sep.:413-24 PMID: 12206879

St Vincent MR, Colpitts CC, Ustinov AV, Muqadas M, Joyce MA, Barsby NL, Epand RF, Epand RM, Khramyshev SA, Valueva OA, Korshun VA, Tyrrell DL, Schang LM. (2010) Rigid amphipathic fusion inhibitors, small molecule antiviral compounds against enveloped viruses. *Proc Natl Acad Sci U S A.* 5; 107(40) Sept.:17339-44. PMID: 20823220

Swallow DL (1977). In: *Progress in Medicinal Chemistry,* G. P. Ellis and G. B. West (eds) Butterworth Group, London, pp. 120.

Verma PC, Basu V, Gupta V, Saxena G, Rahman LU. (2009)Pharmacology and chemistry of a potent hepatoprotective compound Picroliv isolated from the roots and rhizomes of Picrorhiza kurroa royle ex benth. (kutki). *Curr Pharm Biotechnol.* Sep; 10(6):641-9. PMID: 19619118

Wang HM, Liang PH (2010) Picornaviral 3C protease inhibitors and the dual 3C protease/coronaviral 3C-like protease inhibitors. *Expert Opin Ther Pat.*; 20(1) Jan: 59-71. PMID: 20021285

Wen He, Huamin Han, Wei Wang and Bin Gao. (2011) Anti-influenza virus effect of aqueous extracts from dandelion *Virol J.* 14; 8 Dec: 538. PMCID: PMC3265450

Wolf MC, Freiberg AN, Zhang T, Akyol-Ataman Z, Grock A, Hong PW, Li J, Watson NF, Fang AQ, Aguilar HC, Porotto M, Honko AN, Damoiseaux R, Miller JP, Woodson SE, Chantasirivisal S, Fontanes V, Negrete OA, Krogstad P, Dasgupta A, Moscona A,

Hensley LE, Whelan SP, Faull KF, Holbrook MR, Jung ME, Lee B. (2010)A broad-spectrum antiviral targeting entry of enveloped viruses. *Proc Natl Acad Sci U S A* 16; 107(7) Feb: 3157-62

Zhao SS, Tang LH, Fan XG, Chen LZ, Zhou R, Dai X: (2010) Comparison of the efficacy of lamivudine and telbivudine in the treatment of chronic hepatitis B: a systematic review *Virol J*, Sep 3;7:211 PMID:20815890

Zhao SS, Tang LH, Dai XH, Wang W, Zhou R, Chen LZ and Fan XG. (2011)Comparison of the efficacy of tenofovir and adefovir in the treatment of chronic hepatitis B: A Systematic Review *Virology Journal*, 9(8) Mar: 111

ZhuYM, Wang YF, Zhang MY, Zhu L, Kang YY, Men XY, Chen YZ. (2006)The study on the extraction and the antivirus activity of amylase extracted from Grateloupia filicina. *Zhong Yao Cai*: 29(3):256-259.